*the*
# ART
*of*
# SPIRITUAL HEALING

# About the Author

Keith Sherwood was born in New York in 1949. He is an internationally recognized energy master, teacher, and healer, and he lectures and teaches throughout the world and has appeared on many radio and television shows in the United States, Europe, and South Africa.

He is the author of several books on energy work, healing, and transcendent relationships. The exercises, mudras, and meditations that he has developed are used throughout Europe and North America by healers and energy practitioners to heal physical disease, deep traumas, karmic wounds, and energetic blockages. His ability to see and analyze subtle energy fields has been instrumental in helping people achieve their spiritual goals.

Visit Mr. Sherwood on the web at www.onewholelove.com and on Facebook at Keith Sherwood—Onewholelove.

# KEITH SHERWOOD

## *the*
# ART
## *of*
# SPIRITUAL
# HEALING

## CHAKRA AND ENERGY BODYWORK

Llewellyn Publications
Woodbury, Minnesota

SECOND EDITION
First Printing, 2016

Cover art: iStockphoto.com/62314312/©shoo_arts
　　　　　iStockphoto.com/52290746/©HelenStocker
　　　　　iStockphoto.com/4555677/©DNY59
Cover design: Ellen Lawson
Editing: Stephanie Finne
Interior illustrations on pages 15, 50, 67, 71, 78, 88, 102, 138–139, 177, and 218 by
　　Mary Ann Zapalac, all other art by the Llewellyn Art Department. Part page art
　　by iStockphoto.com/62314312/©shoo_arts
Interior photographs provided by Keith Sherwood

Llewellyn Publications is a registered trademark of Llewellyn Worldwide Ltd.

**Library of Congress Cataloging-in-Publication Data**
Sherwood, Keith.
　The art of spiritual healing : chakra and energy bodywork / by Keith Sherwood. --
Updated and Expanded Second Edition.
　　pages cm
　Includes bibliographical references and index.
　ISBN 978-0-7387-4660-9
1.　Spiritual healing.　I. Title.
　BL65.M4S47 2016
　615.8'52—dc23
　　　　　　　　　　　　　　　2015015228

Llewellyn Publications
A Division of Llewellyn Worldwide Ltd.
2143 Wooddale Drive
Woodbury, MN 55125-2989
www.llewellyn.com

Printed in the United States of America

## Other Books by Keith Sherwood

*Chakra Therapy*

*Chakra Healing and Karmic Awareness*

*Energy Healing for Women*

*Sex and Transcendence*

*Die Kunst der Spirituellen Liebe*

*Liebe & Transzendenz*

*Im Bett mit Shiva*

# Contents

## Part 4: Restoring Wellness

# Exercises

# Illustrations

## Introduction

# What You Will Learn

My work with groups and individuals has taught me that what most people want is an easy-to-use book that will provide them with everything they need to perform healing on themselves and other people. *The Art of Spiritual Healing* has been revised to meet those needs and more. You don't have to have any experience with energy work or healing to benefit from it. It's the perfect book for anyone ready and willing to embrace the healing energy and consciousness they have in abundance and use it to restore their body, soul, and spirit to a level of radiant good health.

I wrote the original edition of *The Art of Spiritual Healing* more than thirty years ago and it has helped people in more than twenty-five countries to perform healing safely and effectively. However, since that time much has changed. As a result, I have expanded the scope of the original book beyond healing physical disease. The revised edition includes chapters on healing energetic traumas as well as chapters devoted to healing relationships and maintaining wellness in an ever more complex and stressful world. I've also streamlined and simplified many of the original healing techniques to make them more accessible to people seeking to heal themselves, their relationships, and their clients.

The revised edition of *The Art of Spiritual Healing* has been divided into four parts. In part one, you will learn how to use healing energy and consciousness to help those in need. You will also learn to center yourself in your strong center in your physical body and subtle field. You may not be aware of it, but every human being has a subtle field that interpenetrates their physical body. This field—and the energy and consciousness radiating through it—plays a vital part in maintaining good health and healing disease.

In addition to finding your strong centers, you will learn to see and feel your auric field. You will also use remote viewing and auric assessment to make a health assessment of the disease and/or karmic pattern you wish to heal.

In part two, you will learn the techniques of prana healing, auric healing, and chakra healing. You will learn how to activate chakras, center yourself in chakra fields, and fill your chakra fields with healing energy. In advanced chakra healing, you will learn to heal physical ailments that have their root in the subtle field. In the chapters that follow, you will learn to use vibrational healing and empathetic healing along with the techniques of laying on of hands to heal all forms of physical disease.

In part three, you will learn to heal karmic wounds and energetic traumas that can interfere with the normal activities of a person's soul and spirit. And you will learn to locate and release karmic baggage—a form of subtle energy that can trap a person in self-limiting and destructive patterns.

Part four includes exercises and tips to enhance wellness. Exercises have been provided that will enhance your satisfaction and restore your vitality as well as your ability to share and experience pleasure, love, intimacy, and joy.

By learning the techniques of spiritual healing, you will become a vehicle for healing the world. At the same time, healing energy and consciousness will enrich your life and relationships on the levels of body, soul, and spirit.

## Healing

The energy and consciousness necessary to perform spiritual healing are always radiating through you. They're provided in abundance by

Universal Consciousness to anyone who is receptive to them and asks for them with an open heart. In *The Art of Spiritual Healing* you will learn how to recognize these two powerful forces and use them to perform healing on the levels of body, soul, and spirit.

In the Bhagavad Gita we read "the eternal spirit (Universal Consciousness) ... everywhere are its hands and its feet, everywhere it has eyes that see, heads that think and mouths that speak: everywhere it listens; it dwells in all the worlds, it envelops them all."[1]

Spiritual healing can be likened to the renewing process that goes on continually in every healthy human being and strives to keep everyone healthy. The healer's role is to intercede on behalf of the client when the renewing process has been interrupted and good health has been disrupted. The healer acts as an agent to restore health, harmony, and balance on the physical plane as well as the as the subtle planes of energy and consciousness. He or she does this by channeling healing energy and/or consciousness to the parts of the client's subtle field and physical body that need it most.

Unlike other forms of healing (allopathic, homeopathic, chiropractic, etc.) spiritual healing relies on the ability of the healer to channel healing energy and consciousness directly to his client and the client's ability to use them for their own healing. This is largely an unconscious process that uses abilities that are dormant in all people. Medicine today seeks to alter the conditions in the human body so the body can heal itself, but it doesn't understand what healing is or where the energy and consciousness for healing body, soul, and spirit originate.

In contrast, the spiritual healer recognizes that healing is far more than the removal of physical symptoms and the restoration of physical health; it is a return to balance and harmony. There can never be complete physical health unless the total being is healthy and in harmony with both its internal and external environments.

---

1. Shri P. Swami, trans., *The Geeta, The Gospel of the Lord Shri Krishna* (London: Faber & Faber, 1935), 73.

## Total Health

Radiant good health, on the levels of body, soul, and spirit, is the goal of spiritual healing. This goal is not something that is arrived at and then forgotten; healing is a process. A person either moves in the direction of radiant good health or in the direction of disease. It follows that each person must take individual responsibility for his or her own health. That is why in spiritual healing, the client is not seen as the victim of disease. The client's behavior, attitude, and lifestyle are viewed as important factors in promoting and nourishing the disease. As a result, the client is always seen as the central protagonist in his or her own healing and is called upon to remain active rather than passive during the process of spiritual healing.

It also means that there is never room for complacency when it comes to good health because the human situation is never static. There are negative influences in both the physical and subtle environments that push people toward disease, and there are positive influences that push them toward good health. The healer pays attention to these influences and by keeping them in mind strives to alter negativity and replace it with the conditions that support good health. The healer seeks to heal clients on all levels so that balance and harmony are restored.

## The Healer's View of Disease

Spiritual healers treat disease on the levels of body, soul, and spirit. Therefore it's not surprising that spiritual healers have a unique view of health and disease. They don't view them as separate conditions. They view health and disease as opposite poles of the same thing, differing from each other in degree only. Spiritual healers understand that those who are ill have allowed themselves to drift to the negative pole (disease) and now find it impossible to reach the opposite pole (good health) without outside help.

Because they understand that balance and harmony are essential aspects of good health, spiritual healers recognize that diseases are not caused solely by disease-producing microbes. These creatures are not the root cause of disease. The illnesses they seem to cause are really symptoms of deeper problems that have their foundation in a person's subtle field—the field of energy and consciousness that interpenetrates the physical body and surrounds it on all levels of body, soul, and spirit.

## Nourishment

Different traditions have described the anatomy of the subtle field in different ways. Regardless of how it has been described, imbalances and disharmony can originate in any part of it. The root cause of imbalance and disharmony is separation from an essential source of nourishment, either in the form of energy or consciousness. Separation is most acute when human beings become separated from Universal Consciousness—the source of spiritual nourishment.

Universal Consciousness eternally seeks union with its creation and could secure the health and harmony of each individual entity if they recognized that they required spiritual nourishment to maintain good health. But this awareness is usually lacking, and consequently union is easily disrupted. When disruption occurs, the transfer of energy and consciousness will be restricted. Without sufficient life-affirming energy and consciousness flowing though the subtle field and physical body, a person will begin to slide toward the negative pole (disease) because he or she will not be able to neutralize fields of negativity encountered on the various planes of manifestation, including the physical plane.

## The Four Planes

The healer's world teems with life on every level. He or she sees the physical plane and subtle planes as one large ecology of body, soul, and spirit—all held in balance by the ALL, Universal Consciousness.

Different traditions have given different names to the various levels. To simplify things I will divide the universe into four distinct planes in accordance with the Western metaphysical tradition. This tradition is in large part derived from the ancient Hermetic philosophy and corresponds closely to Christian, yogic, and tantric teachings.

The highest level is the level of transcendent consciousness called the spiritual plane. It's where Universal Consciousness first makes contact with a human being. Below the spiritual plane is the level of human or finite consciousness. It's sometimes called the mental plane. Next is the soul plane, the level of emotions and feelings. Lastly, we come to the physical plane, which is the level of physical life and matter. We humans straddle the dimensions, forming a bridge between the spiritual plane and the lowest plane of physical matter.

## Hermetics

The principles of Hermetics are the foundation of spiritual healing as well as the exercises and healing techniques you will learn to perform in the revised edition of *The Art of Spiritual Healing*. Hermetics originated in ancient Egypt. We are told that it was given to mankind by Thoth, the Egyptian god of wisdom the Greeks later called Hermes Trismegistrus. He was hailed from the earliest times as the "Master of Masters." If Hermes did exist, he is truly the father of esoteric wisdom. The details of his life have been lost to us, but one tradition has it that he was a contemporary of Abraham. Perhaps he was the fabled Melchizedek, whom Abraham paid tithes to and whom Jesus was compared to when he was described as "a priest on the order of Melchizedek."[2]

Whatever the truth may be, Hermes gave us a set of teachings that have influenced philosophy and religion ever since. His teachings are contained in a set of axioms that are set down for the modern student most succinctly in *The Kybalion*. From *The Kybalion*, we learn that the entire philosophy hinges on seven simple principles, and the practice of healing in its many forms is most clearly understood in Hermetic terms.

---

2. Heb. 5:6 (KJV).

The first Hermetic axiom states, "The ALL is mind: the Universe is mental."[3] This doesn't mean what we see in the material world is an illusion, what the Hindus call *maya*. When the Hermetist or healer says that everything is mental, he means that the source—the cosmic root of everything animate and inanimate—is infinite creative mind. (Verbalized in Sanskrit as *ohm*).

Humans can experience infinite mind as it manifests in their spirit by being sentient and self-aware through Universal Consciousness, which is at the center of their being.

The second Hermetic axiom states, "As above, so below; as below, so above."[4] There are planes above us—higher dimensions—that would be beyond our understanding (hidden behind the veils) if the second Hermetic axiom, the Principle of Correspondence, didn't have universal application. Because the Principle of Correspondence applies to all levels at all times, humans can begin to understand the higher planes by studying the lower ones. For the spiritual healer it also means that the same personal resources and techniques can be used to perform healing on the levels of body, soul, and spirit.

The third Hermetic axiom, the Principle of Vibration, states that "nothing rests; everything moves; everything vibrates."[5]

Applying the Principle of Vibration to healing, we can see that not only does everything composed of energy and matter vibrate, but all fields of energy and matter that vibrate have a characteristic rate of vibration that are their unique marks. This means that fields of energy that are part of a person's subtle field can be influenced negatively or positively by other fields they interact with in either their physical or subtle environment. When a person's vibration is negatively affected, disease results.

The process of healing is the process of correcting a person's rate of vibration. We can illustrate this by thinking of disease as a wobble or an unrhythmic vibration. In a car when the tires are poorly aligned, a

---

3. Three Initiates, *The Kybalion: Hermetic Philosophy* (Chicago: Yoga Pub. Soc., 1912), 26.

4. Ibid., 28.

5. Ibid., 30.

wobble develops that affects the steering. To correct it, a person must have the alignment checked and then have the wheels balanced. Once the wobble develops, its uncharacteristic vibration can adversely affect other systems in the car; the same thing can occur in the subtle field. Disease in one area can create disease in a related area or in a nearby system. A wobble also can begin on one level and can be transmuted to the level adjacent to it. For example, an unrhythmic vibration on the level of the soul, if not corrected, will cause damage to both the mental plane and the physical plane.

The fourth Hermetic axiom is called the Principle of Polarity. It states that "everything is dual; everything has poles; everything has its pair of opposites; like and unlike are the same; opposites are identical in nature, but different in degree; extremes meet; all truths are but half truths; all paradoxes may be reconciled."[6] From this principle we can deduce that spirit and matter are simply two poles of the same thing, and everything between them has elements of both, varying from each other only in degree (i.e., vibration). If opposites are really the same and if spirit and matter are the same thing (differing only in their rate of vibration), then they are transmutable and healing energy and/or consciousness (in the form of bliss) can positively affect anything in the physical world, including the physical body. It follows in the human experience that hate can be transmuted into love; pain into joy; disease into perfect health. Because the healer understands the Principle of Polarity, he or she can transmute negative energy into positive, life-affirming energy on every level.

The fifth Hermetic axiom states that "everything flows out and in; everything has its tides; all things rise and fall; the pendulum swing manifests in everything; the measure of the swing to the right is the measure of the swing to the left; rhythm compensates."[7]

The healer understands the law of rhythm and becomes attentive to the natural rhythms he or she finds everywhere, especially those within

---

6. Three Initiates, *The Kybalion*, 32.

7. Ibid., 35.

him- or herself. He or she learns that rhythm compensates and like the great physician Hippocrates said, "Opposites are cures for opposites."[8]

By becoming attentive to his own rhythms and his client's rhythms, the healer can see the wobble in any particular rhythm and can transmute healing energy into the exact vibration or dosage that will compensate for the disease or wobble he finds in his client.

The sixth Hermetic axiom states that "every cause has its effect; every effect has its cause; everything happens according to the law; chance is but a name for law not recognized; there are many planes of causation, but nothing escapes the law."[9] The most important feature of this principle in healing is that nothing happens by chance—the root of every disease is a chain of events that the ill person participated in, even if his participation was largely unconscious. In the final tally he or she is responsible, and as a result he or she will eventually pay the price for past actions through present disease and pain. This law of cause and effect is called karma. In the Book of Galatians the apostle Paul tells us, "... God is not mocked, for whatever a man soweth, that he shall also reap."[10]

The seventh Hermetic axiom is the Principle of Gender. It states that "gender is in everything; everything has its masculine and feminine principles; gender manifests on all planes."[11] Gender, it should be understood, represents far more than sex—the differences between male and female that are quite clear to us on the physical plane. Gender manifests on all planes. On the mental plane, the masculine principle of gender is manifest as the objective mind, the conscious, active mind. The feminine aspect corresponds to the subjective, unconscious, passive mind. On the emotional plane, the masculine principle manifests itself as assertiveness, anger, and all extroverted emotions. The feminine principle manifests itself as receptivity, protection, and

---

8. Hippocrates, *Breaths, Book One [Liber de flatibus]* (Parisiis: Apud Aegidium Gorbinum, 1557), 229.

9. Three Initiates, *The Kybalion*, 38.

10. Isa. 6:13–14 (KJV).

11. Three Initiates, *The Kybalion*, 39.

all introverted emotions. This duality is inherent in all living things, including human beings. As humans, we have within us the masculine assertive element and the feminine receptive element. It is the healer's job to integrate this dual nature first within him- or herself and then within his or her client; to bring everyone he or she works with into harmony and balance.

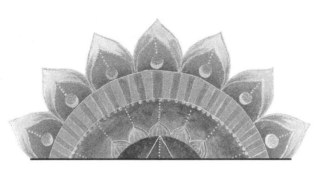

## Part 1

# Introduction to Spiritual Healing and Analysis

# Chapter 1
# Healing Energy and Consciousness

Healing energy and consciousness are so powerful that when they radiate through you freely they can catapult you into a state of transcendence. In this state, disease disappears and you can participate in the pleasure, love, intimacy, and joy that is continuously experienced by the living universe.

The consciousness I'm talking about is called bliss. The energy I'm talking about goes by many names and has been venerated in many societies. Taoists in China call it *chi* or *ki*. In India, it's called *prana* and *shakti*. It doesn't matter what name it goes by—this extraordinary energy, like bliss, only has universal qualities, which means it can be used to heal physical disease, energetic traumas, and karmic patterns that have restricted your access to the power, creativity, and radiance that is your birthright.

Universal qualities of this energy include vitality, creativity, and the power to heal as well as pleasure, love, intimacy, joy, and the qualities of good character—which for millennia have been embraced by healers of all cultures. Knowing yourself as an expression of these universal qualities will empower you to become an agent of healing wherever you go.

## The Subtle Field of Energy and Consciousness

In spiritual healing, you will be working primarily with resources lying dormant within your subtle field of energy and consciousness.

This may sound strange to those of you who are new to spiritual healing. But spiritual masters and healers have recognized for millennium that people are interdimensional beings who exists, interact, and function in both the physical world and the subtle world of energy and consciousness. In practice this means that you have both a physical body and a subtle field of consciousness and prana (non-physical energy) that interpenetrates your physical body. The remarkable field of consciousness and energy, that I call the subtle field, contains non-physical vehicles. These vehicles coordinate their activities with your physical body so that you can express yourself freely and participate fully in both the physical and non-physical universe.

Although most people are unaware of their existence, subtle vehicles are responsible for maintaining health and well-being and for providing human beings with the ability to form an authentic identity and participate joyfully in all the activities associated with life on Earth. In addition to these vehicles, the subtle field contains resource fields and a subtle energy system.

Resource fields are vast fields of prana and consciousness that interpenetrate your subtle field. They're the largest parts of your subtle field and function as a link between each individual human being and the source of healing, Universal Consciousness. Resource fields nourish your vehicles of energy and consciousness as well as the other organs of your subtle field (chakras, meridians, auras, etc.), and they provide you with the prana and consciousness you need to perform healing on the levels of body, soul, and spirit.

The subtle energy system includes chakras and chakra fields, meridians, auric fields, and minor energy centers scattered throughout your subtle energy system.

Chakras are vortices that transmit prana through your subtle field. Everybody has 146 chakras that correspond to the 146 dimensions within the physical and non-physical universe. The thirteen most important chakras are located in your body space (the space in the non-physical universe that interpenetrates your physical body).

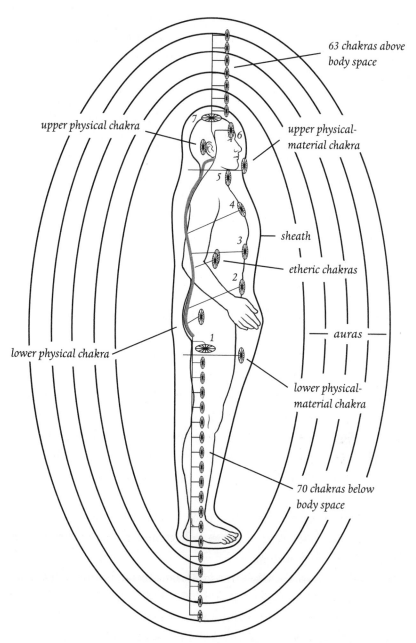

63 chakras above
body space

upper physical chakra

upper physical-
material chakra

sheath

etheric chakras

auras

lower physical chakra

lower physical-
material chakra

70 chakras below
body space

*The Subtle Field of Energy and Consciousness*

Meridians are streams of energy that connect your chakras to your subtle fields and physical body. There are ten ruling meridians and thousands of lesser meridians scattered throughout your subtle fields.

Auric fields are egg-shaped fields of prana and consciousness that surround your subtle vehicles on all physical and non-physical dimensions. They have two parts: an inner cavity that serves as a reservoir of prana and consciousness and a surface boundary that separates your internal environment from the external environment.

Minor energy centers are centers of energetic activity scattered through your subtle field. The most important minor energy centers are located in your hands and feet. Minor energy centers support your chakras and meridians by facilitating the movement of prana through your subtle fields and physical body.

In the pages that follow, we will look more deeply at both your subtle field and subtle energy system. For now, it's important to know two things. First, in the same way that an electrical grid provides energy to homes and businesses, your resource fields and the organs of your subtle energy system (chakras, meridians, auric field, and minor energy centers) transmit all the energy and consciousness your subtle vehicles and physical body need to function healthfully and to perform healing on the levels of body, soul, and spirit.

Second, to benefit from all the consciousness and healing energy you have available—and to radiate them both effectively—it's necessary to find your strong center in your physical body and subtle field.

## Finding Your Strong Center

Your strong center in your physical body brings your awareness back inside your body space where it belongs (body space is the space occupied by your physical body on the physical plane and your subtle vehicles on the subtle planes). Your strong center in your subtle field takes you out of the past and future and keeps you firmly centered in the ever-present Now, the only place where spiritual healing can take place. By integrating your two strong centers, you will become a channel for healing yourself and the world.

Tantric and Taoist adepts were among the first to recognize the importance of remaining centered in both strong centers. They taught their students that if their awareness remained ahead of their physical body and subtle vehicles while performing healing, they would fall out of the ever-present Now and position themselves in the future. And if their awareness remained behind their subtle field and physical body while performing healing, they would fall out of the ever-present Now and position themselves in the past. These initial insights confirmed to the Tantrists and Taoists that to perform healing effectively it was essential to be centered squarely in both physical and subtle strong centers because healing always took place in the ever-present Now.

You can reclaim your strong center, first in your physical body by centering yourself in *Hara* and then in your subtle field by performing the *standard method*. Then you can integrate their functions by using the *prana integration mudra*. The prana integration mudra will integrate the flow of energy and consciousness that connects them both and it will keep you centered and strong.

### Physical Center (The Hara)

The Hara is located four fingers' width below your navel and about one inch (2.5 cm) forward from your spine. In Japanese, the word *Hara* means "abdomen." Hara is often linked with another Japanese word *tanden*. *Tanden* means "elixir field." Hara can therefore be understood to be the place in your physical body where you can find the elixir of life. It is also the place where you can reclaim your strong center in your physical body.

Most people in the West are unaware of the importance of Hara. That is one reason why so many people still lack all the vitality and healing power available to them. It also explains why so many people are out of balance and why they're suspended from a point just above their shoulders and dangle there like puppets. Their physical body and its posture reflect the fact that they have not made Hara a part of their everyday lives.

Problems such as poor posture, chronic muscle tension that inhibits the flow of prana through the subtle field, compressed and twisted spine, cramped body organs, and poor circulation can be directly linked to being balanced from the shoulders instead of from Hara.

Not being centered in your strong center in your physical body can create additional problems. It can put strain on the joints and ligaments. And that can contribute to mental and physical fatigue—even depression.

So, what is to be gained by Hara? A great deal. Reclaiming your strong center in Hara will empower you by drawing your awareness back inside your physical body. It will connect the centers of energy and consciousness in your abdomen with those in your heart and head. Your reproductive organs will receive more nourishment and will function better. And, by liberating the energy in your abdomen, you will have greater access to your deepest emotions and feelings.

The simplest way to reclaim your strong center in Hara is by practicing a technique called *Hara breathing*.

---

### Exercise: Hara Breathing

Hara breathing is an ancient technique that has been practiced in the Far East for centuries. It's designed to help people find their strong center in their physical body and to integrate the functions of their physical body with one another. If you feel alienated from your body or empty and in need of inner strength, agitated or overwhelmed, scared or angry, breathing into the Hara will bring you relief.

You can practice Hara breathing in any position as long as your back is straight. For now, I suggest you perform Hara breathing while you're lying down on your back. As you progress, you can practice the exercise in a sitting or standing position.

It's best to begin Hara breathing with your arms at your sides, palms up, and your fingers loosely extended. Your eyes should be closed and your jaw kept loose by allowing your mouth to drop open comfortably. From this position, you will begin breathing deeply through your nose for about three to four minutes. Then you will shift your mental attention to your Hara, which is four finger widths below your navel.

Once you've brought your mental attention to Hara, the first thing you'll notice is a vibration. A short time later, you'll experience sensations emerging from this vital point. You could experience warmth, tingling and/or throbbing sensations, coolness, or pressure. None of these sensations should worry you; they're all normal.

It's important to note that a significant source of prana is your breath. Prana enters your subtle field on each inhalation. Prana vibrates and once it interacts with Hara, it will cause a sympathetic vibration that will activate it further.

Continue to breathe deeply through your nose for two to three minutes. After two to three minutes, inhale through your nose for a count of five. As you inhale, feel that you're breathing into Hara. To enhance the effect, visualize that a fluid is flowing in and filling that vital point with energy and light. Retain your breath for a count of five while your mental attention remains focused on Hara. During the retention, you will begin to feel your Hara heating up and your center of balance shifting to that vital point.

After you've retained the breath for a count of five, exhale through your mouth for a count of five. There should be no separation between exhalation and the next inhalation. Only in the retention is the natural rhythm broken.

Perform this exercise two to three times a week for about twenty minutes. By mastering Hara breathing, you will return to your strong center in your physical body. And you will enhance the energy you have available for healing. Repeat as needed.

## Subtle Energy Center

Now that you've learned to center yourself in Hara, you're ready to reclaim your strong center in your subtle field. To do that, you will perform an exercise called the standard method. The standard method takes about twenty minutes. In the first part, you will relax the major muscle groups of your physical body by contracting and releasing them. This helps to quiet your mind by releasing residual stress and energy stored in tense muscles. In the second part, you will use your intent to center yourself in your subtle field.

It's important to note that in this exercise your intent serves the same function as a computer software program. Just as a software program instructs a computer to perform a particular task, your intent instructs your authentic mind to turn your organs of perception inward.

Your organs of perception include your senses, which gather physical input, as well as your other, non-physical means of knowing, such as intuition. If you use your intent properly—without watching yourself, trying too hard, or mixing your intent with sentiment and self-doubt—your perception will automatically turn inward.

---

### Exercise: The Standard Method

To begin the standard method, find a comfortable position with your back straight. Close your eyes and breathe deeply through your nose for two to three minutes. Then slowly count backward from five to one. As you count backward, mentally repeat and visualize each number three times to yourself. Take your time and let your mind be as creative as it likes. Continue by counting backward from ten to one, letting yourself sink deeper on each descending number.

Next, inhale and bring your attention to your feet. Contract the muscles of your feet as much as possible. Hold your breath for five seconds. Then release your breath and allow the muscles of your feet to relax. Inhale deeply again and repeat the process with your ankles and calves. Continue in the same way with your knees, thighs, buttocks and pelvis, middle and upper abdomen, chest, shoulders, neck, arms, and hands.

After you've tightened and relaxed all those body parts, squeeze the muscles of your face and hold for five seconds. After five seconds, release and say *ahh* as you exhale. Next, open your mouth, stick out your tongue, and stretch the muscles of your face as much as possible. Hold for five seconds. Then release the muscles of your face and say *ahh* as you exhale.

Finally, contract your entire body and squeeze the muscles of your face while you hold your breath for five seconds. Expel the breath through your nose and relax for a few moments.

When you're ready to continue, assert, "*It's my intent to center myself in my subtle field of energy and consciousness.*" Take a few moments to enjoy the effects; then assert, "*It's my intent to turn my organs of perception* (your organs of perception include your eyes, ears, nose, the nerve endings in your body that produce sensation, and your intuition) *inward on the levels of my subtle field.*"

Immediately your orientation will shift, and from your new vantage point deep within yourself you will become aware that you're centered in your subtle field because you will feel lighter, more yourself, and, most importantly, thoughts and feelings will no longer distract you.

Take fifteen minutes more to enjoy the exercise. Then count from one to five and open your eyes. The more often you use the standard method, the greater the benefits will be and the easier it will be to stay centered in your subtle field without being distracted.

## Integrating and Balancing Your Strong Centers

Now that you've learned to center yourself in your strong center in your physical body and subtle field, you can integrate and balance their functions. To do that, you will use a mudra specifically designed for that purpose. It's called the prana integration mudra.

A mudra is a symbolic gesture that can be made with the hands and fingers or in combination with the tongue and feet. The word *mudra* comes from the Sanskrit root *mud*, which means "delight or pleasure."

Although new to the Western world, mudras have been used in the East for centuries to enhance physical, mental, emotional, and spiritual well-being. Taoists in ancient China used them to find inner peace;

Indian mystics used them to attain samadhi (enlightenment); and healers have used them to heal everything from headaches to arthritis.

Mudras work because they stimulate the flow of healing energy, prana/chi, through specific energetic centers in the subtle energy system. By stimulating these points for extended periods of time, usually for five minutes or more, it's possible to both enhance and integrate the flow of prana between the subtle field and the physical body.

In the next exercise, you will learn to perform the prana integration mudra. After that, you will use it along with Hara breathing and the standard method to integrate and balance your strong center in your physical body and subtle field.

---

### Exercise: The Prana Integration Mudra

To perform the prana integration mudra, find a comfortable position with your back straight. Breathe deeply through your nose for two to three minutes. Then close your eyes and place your left thumb into the cavity created by your right thumb and the index finger. Next, place your left index finger over your right middle finger. Continue by placing your left middle finger over your right ring finger and your left ring finger over the right pinky. Once your fingers are in position, bring your tongue to the top of your mouth. Then slide it back until the upper palate becomes soft.

Hold the mudra for ten minutes. Then release it and open your eyes.

By performing the prana integration mudra, you will feel more energy radiating through your physical body and subtle field, especially through the parts that have contracted and need it the most. However, the true value of the prana integration mudra will only become apparent when you combine it with Hara breathing and the standard method in the following exercise.

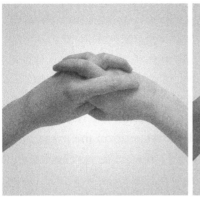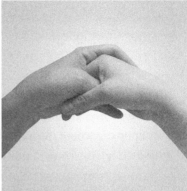

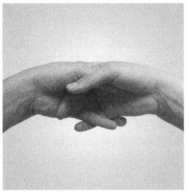

*Three Views of the Prana Integration Mudra*

---

### Exercise: Integrating and Balancing
### Your Strong Centers

In the exercise that follows, you will use the prana integration mudra to integrate and balance the energy radiating from your strong center in Hara and your subtle field.

To begin, find a comfortable position with your back straight. Then close your eyes and center yourself in Hara by performing Hara breathing. Once you're centered in Hara, perform the standard method. Enjoy the shift for two to three minutes. Then perform the prana integration mudra. Hold the mudra for ten minutes while you let thoughts and feelings come and go without interference. In a short time, your mind will become quiet and you will enjoy the refreshing energy that connects your physical body to your subtle field. After ten minutes, release the mudra and breathe normally again. Then count from one to five. When you reach the number five, open your eyes and bring yourself out of the exercise.

If you integrate and balance your strong centers regularly, your appreciation of the non-physical world will grow stronger. So will your discernment and your ability to access the healing energy and consciousness you will need for spiritual healing.

## Summary

In chapter one, you learned about the importance of your subtle field and subtle energy system. You also learned to integrate the functions of your physical body and subtle field by centering yourself in Hara and your subtle field of energy and consciousness. After that, you integrated and balanced the flow of energy between your strong centers by performing the prana integration mudra. Now that you understand the importance of your strong centers, you are ready to enhance your innate healing skills so that you become a more effective healer.

# Chapter 2
# Enhancing Your Healing Skills

Knowledge, personal resources, and healing power are necessary to become a skilled and effective healer. The personal resources I'm referring to include your intent, mental attention, prana, and transcendental consciousness in the form of bliss. It's by combining these resources in the appropriate way that you will be able to locate concentrations of distorted energy and consciousness and heal the diseases they create.

## The Authentic Mind

All the resources you will be using have their foundation in your subtle field. But they emerge into your conscious awareness through your authentic mind.

Your authentic mind is the vehicle through which you manifest and focus your authentic identity and the functions of mind that support it—intent, will, desire, resistance, etc.—into the world around you. It emerged from Universal Consciousness through the tattvas. The word *tattva* comes from the Sanskrit root words *tat*, which means "that," and *tvam*, which means "thou" or "you." As evolution proceeded, via the tattvas, a hierarchy of physical and non-physical dimensions was created in both the physical and non-physical universe. You exist on all of these dimensions. And on all of these dimensions, your mind has the capacity to use prana and consciousness to perform spiritual healing.

Though it's designed to function as a unified whole, your authentic mind is divided into three essential parts: On the physical level, your authentic mind is the brain, the nervous system, and the chemicals in the body, including hormones that influence its structure and activities.

On the non-physical level, your authentic mind includes your subtle field of energy and consciousness, its organs and vehicles, and the consciousness and prana that nourish them.

The combination of physical and non-physical elements creates the third part of the human mind—the network. The network includes the connections the mind has to its individual parts and to things beyond itself. This includes consciousness and energy as well as connections to other people, non-physical beings, and their projections. It's the existence of a network that explains how the healer can make contact with his client on non-physical dimensions and how the prana and consciousness the healer projects to the client can heal disease in the client's body, soul, and spirit.

There are three ways that a spiritual healer can use the network to make contact with a client in need of healing. A spiritual healer can use energetic vehicles, known as sheaths, within their own subtle field to make contact. Sheaths have the ability to extend themselves vast distances and to channel healing energy and consciousness. A spiritual healer can use chakras, using the subtle energy system to radiate healing energy to a client. Finally, he or she can use the organs of perception, particularly the eyes, to make direct contact.

The organs of perception (eyes, ears, nose, etc.) are also part of the human mind. They can be directed inward into the mind itself or outward into the external environment. When they're directed outward, they can make contact with other networks and interact with them.

## Functions of Mind

Although the human mind can be directed both inward and outward—and it can change disease into health—it still has a limited number of functions or ways it can interact with its environment. The ways it can interact are known as its functions of mind. For more than thirty years I've studied the interactions the subtle field and network can have with its physical and subtle environment. In that time, I've learned that there are sixteen functions of mind. They include intent, will, desire, resistance, surrender, acceptance, knowing, choice, commitment, rejection, faith, enjoyment, destruction, creativity, empathy, and love. In spiritual healing, your intent plays a unique role, which is why you will be using it in most of the diagnostic and healing techniques you will learn in the following pages.

### *Intent*

In spiritual healing, your intent serves the same function as a computer software program. Just as a software program instructs a computer to perform a particular task, your intent can instruct your authentic mind to use the consciousness and energy it has in abundance to heal disease in body, soul, and/or spirit. If you use your intent properly—without watching yourself, trying too hard, or mixing your intent with sentiment and self-doubt—it will become a valuable skill that will be part of virtually all the healing techniques you perform in this book.

Intent is one of sixteen functions of mind located within a resource field called the core field. Resource fields, such as the core field, are extremely large fields of prana and consciousness that interpenetrate your subtle field and provide it with the nourishment it needs to function healthfully.

In order to enhance the clarity of your intent and make it an effective tool for healing, you will perform an exercise called the *enhanced intent meditation*. In the enhanced intent meditation, you will experience your intent as part of a large field of consciousness and energy that is free of energetic attachments or fields of distorted energy.

---

### Exercise: Enhanced Intent Meditation

To begin the enhanced intent meditation, find a comfortable position with your back straight. Close your eyes and breathe deeply through your nose for two to three minutes. Then count backward from five to one and from ten to one. Use the standard method to relax your muscles and to center yourself in your subtle field of energy and consciousness. Then assert, "*It's my intent to center myself in my core field.*" Take a few moments to enjoy the shift. Then assert, "*It's my intent to shift my center to the portion of my core field associated with intent.*"

Continue by asserting, "*It's my intent to turn my organs of perception inward on the portion of my core field associated with intent.*" Next, assert, "*It's my intent to enhance the clarity and strength of my intent.*" Take fifteen minutes to enjoy the process. During that time don't try to control your thoughts and feelings or use visualization as a meditation aid. You will receive more benefits from the exercise if you give up all striving and let the exercise lead you into a deeper recognition of the power and significance of your intent.

After fifteen minutes, bring yourself out of the meditation by counting from one to five. When you reach the number five, open your eyes. You will feel wide awake, perfectly relaxed, and better than you did before. You only need to perform this exercise once.

Now that you have enhanced the clarity and strength of your intent you can use it to instruct your mental attention to perform whatever diagnostic and healing activities you have in mind.

## Mental Attention

By using your mental attention skillfully, you can heal ailments in body, soul, and spirit. That's because your mental attention functions simultaneously on all worlds and dimensions in both the physical and non-physical universe. With intent as a guide, your mental attention can be used to visualize the condition of a person's subtle field and physical body. Then it can be used to create new realities of radiant good health to replace the conditional reality of disease.

In the exercise that follows, you will use your mental attention, along with your intent, to create a visual screen. You can use your visual screen to view an image of yourself or another person. Once an image has appeared on your screen, you can use your mental attention to diagnose and heal disease in your subject's physical body and/or soul and spirit. The screen you create should be eight feet (2.5 m) in front of you, white, and large enough to fit a life-size image of a person. It should be raised off the floor so that you must look up at a thirty-degree angle to see the image on the screen clearly.

---

## Exercise: The Visual Screen

To use your intent and mental attention to create a visual screen, find a comfortable position with your back straight. Close your eyes and breathe deeply through your nose for two to three minutes. Then count backward from five to one and from ten to one. Use the standard method to relax your muscles and to center yourself in your subtle field of energy and consciousness.

When you're ready to continue, assert, *"It's my intent to create a white screen eight feet (2.5 m) in front of me."* Once the visual screen has materialized, assert, *"It's my intent to visualize an image of myself on the screen."* Immediately, you will see an image of yourself appear on the screen in a size to fit comfortably. Observe it for about five minutes. After five minutes, release the image of yourself and the visual screen. Then count from one to five. When you reach the number five, open your eyes and bring yourself out of the meditation.

If you have any difficulty seeing and feeling the image of yourself on the screen, practice the exercise every day for a week. It's not necessary to see every part of your body with perfect clarity to diagnose and heal disease. Therefore, there is no need to worry if you weren't completely successful. Your ability to see images on the screen will increase dramatically with practice.

## Energy with Universal Qualities

To enhance the flow of prana through your energy field so that you have all the prana you need for healing, you will perform the *prana mudra*.

## Exercise: The Prana Mudra

To perform the prana mudra, find a comfortable position with your back straight. Breathe deeply through your nose for two to three minutes. Then use the standard method to relax your muscles and center yourself in your subtle field of energy and consciousness.

When you're ready to continue, bring the tip of your tongue to the point where the inside of your gums meets your upper teeth. Then bring the tip of your thumbs to the inside of the first joint of your index fingers so that they form two loops.

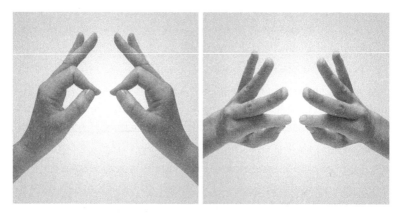

*The Prana Mudra*

Hold the mudra for ten minutes, with your eyes closed, while you allow prana to radiate through your subtle field and physical body. Don't do anything more while you hold the mudra. You will receive more benefits from it if you give up all striving and let the prana mudra lead you into a deeper experience of your innate strength and healing power.

After ten minutes, release the mudra and count from one to five. When you reach the number five, open your eyes and bring yourself out of the exercise. By repeating the prana mudra regularly you will raise your energetic level to new heights.

This will enhance your vitality and make more healing energy available for self-healing and healing other people.

## Orgasmic Bliss

Orgasmic bliss is the most powerful force in the universe. Every human being is in bliss, although most people are unaware of it. According to the Tantrists, orgasmic bliss is an enduring condition, deep inside your subtle field, created through the union of consciousness (Shiva) and energy (Shakti).

It's important to note that bliss is not a form of energy. Rather, it is the highest form of consciousness that radiates through your subtle field and physical body. The merging of consciousness and energy with universal qualities provides you with a constant flow of healing power that can heal even the densest concentrations of distorted subtle energy.

To use orgasmic bliss to heal disease, you must bring it into your conscious awareness and keep it there during the healing process. That's because you must radiate bliss consciously in order to heal yourself or to heal another person.

To bring bliss into your conscious awareness, you will learn to perform a mudra specifically designed for that purpose. The mudra is called the *orgasmic bliss mudra*.

---

### Exercise: The Orgasmic Bliss Mudra

To perform the orgasmic bliss mudra, find a comfortable position with your back straight. Breathe deeply through your nose for two to three minutes. Use the standard method to relax your muscles and to center yourself in your subtle field of energy and consciousness. Then place the tip of your tongue on your upper palette and bring it straight back until it comes to rest at the point where the hard palette rolls up and becomes soft.

Once the tip of your tongue is in that position, put the bottom of your feet together so that the soles are touching. Then bring your hands in front of your solar plexus and place the inside tips of your thumbs together. Continue by bringing the outside of your index fingers together from the tips to the first joint. Next, bring the outside of your middle fingers together from the first to the second joint. The fourth and fifth fingers should be curled into your palm.

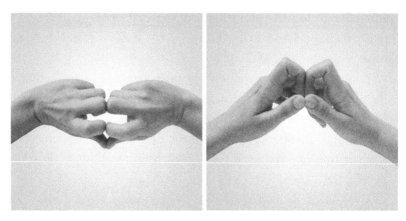

*The Orgasmic Bliss Mudra*

Once your tongue, fingers, and feet are in position, close your eyes and breathe through your nose. Hold the mudra for ten minutes. Then release your fingers, separate the soles of your feet, and bring your tongue back to its normal position. Next, count from one to five. When you reach the number five, open your eyes. You will be wide awake and perfectly relaxed, and you'll feel better than you did before.

## Summary

In this chapter, you learned how to enhance the resources you will use in spiritual healing. Those resources include intent, mental attention, and healing energy in the form of prana and bliss. By practicing the exercises you learned regularly, you will be handsomely rewarded. Your confidence as a healer will grow and you will build a lasting foundation that will enable you to radiate more healing energy and consciousness to people who need it.

In the following chapter, you will learn to discern the difference between healing energy and energy that causes disease. Then you will learn to use your intent, mental attention, and healing energy in the form of prana to perform remote viewing in the mineral, vegetable, and animal kingdoms. Remote viewing is a diagnostic tool that will provide you with the information you need on both the subtle and physical levels to successfully perform spiritual healing.

# Chapter 3

# Remote Viewing and Assessment

In the last two chapters, you found your strong center in your physical body and subtle energy field and you've enhanced your healing skills by performing the exercises and mudras. So, it shouldn't surprise you to learn that spiritual healers have a unique view of health and disease. One reason for their unique view is that they rely on their discernment, which is a function of the inductive mind to diagnose disease.

The inductive mind uses intuition and insight to gain knowledge of the world. Discernment, which is a precise form of intuition, is the ability to see, feel, and/or sense fields of non-physical energy. With enhanced discernment, a healer can see and feel diseased energy in their client's subtle field. That's because the subtle fields of energy and consciousness that support good health only have universal qualities, while the fields that support disease have individual qualities, which means they look, feel, and vibrate differently.

Universal qualities are life affirming. They not only support good health, they support wellness by bringing people together in the most direct and joyful ways possible—for example, pleasure, love, intimacy, joy, truth, freedom, and unconditional love. Universal qualities don't cause attachment and bind people to each other in unhealthy ways either. Rather, universal qualities—and the consciousness and energy that support them—enhance freedom, self-awareness, and the state of transcendence where problems and worries disappear and you can participate in the bliss that is continuously experienced by the living universe.

## Energy with Individual Qualities

The energy that causes disease has individual qualities. It has what we can call a flavor. You already know this energy. It's the same dense energy that creates pressure and muscle ache when you're stressed and produces anxiety, self-doubt, and confusion when it's consciously or unconsciously activated. In fact, energy with individual qualities in one form or another is the principal source of both human suffering and physical disease. When energy with individual qualities accumulates in your subtle energy field, it can create blockages. It does that by disrupting the flow of prana through your chakras, meridians, and minor energy centers.

A field of energy with individual qualities, such as the subtle fields that cause depression and anxiety or that press on you from the outside, can look like a wave or small pool of dense energy that is active and can move, especially when you bring your attention to it. Because of its density and its ability to move, it can block prana the same way dirt can block the flow of clean air through an air filter.

It's these blockages that cause disease on the physical level and self-limiting and destructive patterns on the levels of soul and spirit. Many of these blockages have been with you for lifetimes, since you carry the energy that supports them in your subtle field from one incarnation to the next.

It's because the healer can discern the difference between healing energy and the distorted energy that he or she doesn't see disease and health as separate conditions. Nor does he or she believe that microbes are the ultimate cause of most diseases. The illnesses microbes seem to cause are really symptoms of deeper problems that can be traced back to a person's subtle field of energy and consciousness.

## Remote Viewing

In the following pages, you will learn to enhance your discernment, turning it from a vague feeling analogous to intuition into a reliable and precise tool that you can use to see and feel subtle fields. By doing that, you will be able to distinguish healthy energy from the energy that causes disease. The first step will be to learn the techniques of remote viewing.

It may surprise you to learn that remote viewing is a relatively simple technique to master. In fact, you're continually practicing remote viewing while dreaming at night and when you're daydreaming or using your imagination. When you're imagining yourself in a particular place or situation, you're actually projecting your mental attention to it on the mental plane, where it's located. Everything that exists on the physical plane had a prior existence on the mental plane before it was transmuted into physical reality. So, don't be confused; when you see spontaneous images, you see things that are real, and that can have a profound effect on your health and well-being.

### Remote Viewing in the Three Kingdoms

In the exercises that follow, you will enhance your discernment by performing remote viewing on the three levels of matter on the physical plane: the mineral kingdom, the vegetable kingdom, and the animal kingdom.

To perform remote viewing, you must first center yourself in your subtle field of energy and consciousness. To do that, you will perform the standard method. After that, you will use your intent along with your mental attention to create a visual screen. It's on your visual screen that you will visualize specimens from the three kingdoms. After studying your specimens from the outside, you will use your intent and mental attention to mentally project yourself inside the specimens so that you can discern their qualities down to the molecular level.

---

### Exercise: Remote Viewing

To begin the exercise, find a comfortable position with your back straight. Then close your eyes and breathe deeply through your nose for two to three minutes. Use the standard method to relax your muscles and to center yourself in your subtle field of energy and consciousness.

When you're ready to continue, assert, *"It's my intent to visualize a white screen eight feet (2.5 m) in front of me."* Once the visual screen has materialized, assert, *"It's my intent to visualize a large, brown stone about one foot (30 cm) in diameter on my visual screen."* Keep your senses open and active as you observe the stone because using the five senses is just as important on the mental plane as it is on the physical plane. Some people mistakenly believe there is a sixth sense that is used exclusively to experience the higher planes. This is not exactly the case. The sixth sense is no more than human intuition, which the healer calls clairsentience. Along with the five senses, the healer uses clairsentience to gather information from the subtle planes of energy and consciousness.

After you've examined the stone from eight feet (2.5 m) away and have observed its size, shape, color, and texture, visualize yourself standing beside it close enough to reach out and touch it. Feel the stone's surface texture, density, temperature, etc. Details are important in the process of assessment, so the more qualities you can experience, the better.

After you've examined the stone from close up, you will adjust your size and project yourself inside. To do that, assert, *"It's my intent to project myself inside the stone in the appropriate size to fit comfortably."* Use all of the appropriate senses to explore the inside of the stone. Use your intuition to feel the spirit of the stone, what you can think of as its essence. All things created have an essence, and by experiencing it, a healer can actually sense the rightness or wrongness of its vibration. Sensing the rightness or wrongness is extremely important in spiritual healing because a sense of wrongness is often the first indication of disease in someone's subtle field of energy and consciousness.

Take three to four minutes to explore the inside of the stone. When you're satisfied that you've experienced the stone in its fullness, visualize yourself standing outside once again, sitting in front of your screen. Then release the stone. Take a deep breath and go deeper (relax more completely).

When you're ready to continue, visualize a pot of tulips on the screen in front of you. Get a sense of the rightness or wrongness of its vibration. Then examine the size, shape, color, and texture of the plant. After two to three minutes, visualize yourself standing next to it, close enough to reach out and touch it. Take a few moments to examine the tulips close up. Then take a deep breath and mentally repeat the affirmation, "*It's my intent to project myself inside the tulip plant in the appropriate size to fit comfortably.*" As soon as you're inside, examine the organs of the flower. Move from the flowers down to the stem and from the stem to the roots. Since you're dealing with a complex living organism, take your time and experience both the physical qualities of the plant and the life force that animates it. The life force is a manifestation of both consciousness and prana.

I suggest you take about five minutes or more to complete your examination of the plant. When you've experienced the plant in its fullness, mentally project yourself back to your original position in front of your visual screen. Then release the plant, take a deep breath, and feel yourself going deeper.

From remote viewing in the vegetable kingdom, you will now move to remote viewing in the animal kingdom. By moving to the animal kingdom, you can make contact with your subject on more levels, including the animal's consciousness, emotions, and feelings.

When you're ready to continue, visualize an animal on your screen. A household pet is your best bet; however, you can visualize any animal you're familiar with—either a farm animal or an animal you've seen at a zoo or in the wild. Once it has appeared on your screen, examine the animal's physical body from top to bottom. After a few moments, visualize yourself standing next to the animal. Reach out and begin stroking it. Be attentive to the creature's reaction. You can learn much about your subject in this way. Continue using all of your senses, but pay special attention to the rightness or wrongness of the animal's vibration.

When you're satisfied with what you've learned, you can continue remote viewing by projecting yourself inside the animal's body by their lungs. To do that, assert, *"It's my intent to mentally project myself inside* (the name of the animal here) *in the appropriate size to fit comfortably."* As soon as you're inside the animal's body, reach out your hand and touch one of its lungs. You will feel the rhythmic movement of the lungs as the animal breathes in and out. Be attentive to the rightness or wrongness of the vibration.

When you've experienced the lungs and the area around them to your satisfaction, move to the base of the animal's spinal column. Reach out and touch one of the vertebrae. Notice the difference between the various organs in the spinal area. Take two to three minutes to examine the vertebra, spinal column, and surrounding organs. After two to three minutes, begin to move freely around the animal's body. If you go to a diseased area, notice the differences between healthy and diseased tissue.

Take another five to ten minutes to complete your examination. Then mentally project yourself back to your seat in front of your visual screen. Release the animal and the visual screen next. Then count from one to five and bring yourself out of the exercise.

Now that you've learned to perform remote viewing in the mineral, vegetable, and animal kingdoms, you're ready to take remote viewing a step further by using it to diagnose disease in a human body. To do that, you will use the techniques of remote viewing to examine your own body and discern its condition.

---

## Exercise: Remote Assessment

To begin the exercise, find a comfortable position with your back straight. Then close your eyes and breathe deeply through your nose for two to three minutes. Use the standard method to relax your muscles and center yourself in your subtle field of energy and consciousness.

When you're ready to continue, assert, "*It's my intent to visualize a white screen eight feet (2.5 m) in front of me.*" Once the visual screen has materialized, assert, "*It's my intent to visualize an image of myself on the screen.*" Once the image appears, examine it for two to three minutes. Pay attention to the different parts of your body and the rightness or wrongness of their vibration. Examine your posture and the expression on your face. If you're attracted to any particular part of your body, it's usually an indication that its vibration has been disrupted. Take note of it and move on.

When you're satisfied with your examination, visualize yourself standing next to the image of yourself on the screen. Scan your body for another minute or two. When you feel satisfied that you've gleaned as much useful information as possible, assert, "*It's my intent to project myself inside my body, standing next to my lungs, in the appropriate size to fit comfortably.*" Instantaneously, you will find yourself standing between your two lungs.

Use all the appropriate senses to examine your lungs. Reach out and touch one of them. Feel the rhythmic movement of the lungs on each inhalation and exhalation. Experience all the physical qualities as well as the rightness or wrongness of their vibration. Ask yourself the question: Are the lungs functioning normally; are they healthy and in harmony? The ability to experience something completely is an acquired skill, so don't be discouraged if you can't experience the lungs in their fullness right away. With practice, you will.

When you've experienced the lungs and the area around them to your satisfaction, project yourself to the base of the spinal column. Reach out and touch one of the vertebrae. Take two to three minutes to examine the vertebra, spinal column, and surrounding tissue. After two to three minutes, project yourself to another part of your body. If you go to a diseased area, notice the differences between healthy and diseased tissue. Continue scanning the inside of your body for five minutes more.

When you're finished, assert, "*It's my intent to return to my original position eight feet (2.5 m) in front of my visual screen.*" Release the image of yourself and the visual screen next. Then count from one to five and bring yourself out of the exercise.

Now that you've learned how to perform remote viewing, you can refine your ability through repetition. Even if you had only limited success, with practice your ability will improve, and in time you will be able to use all of your senses as well as your insight and intuition to diagnose ailments within a person's body and subtle field.

## Symbols and Assessment—A Case History

Sometimes, an ailment in a person's body will appear symbolically rather than objectively. The following case history illustrates what I mean. In a seminar I was conducting, I used remote viewing as part of a case reading. Case readings are one of the best ways I know for practicing remote viewing and assessment. In this case reading, a seminar participant got me permission to perform a health assessment on a friend. Then she wrote the woman's name, age, and address on the outside of a folded piece of paper. On the inside, she wrote down all her friend's medical and psychological ailments. Since the paper was folded, I couldn't see what was written on the inside. Then she guided me into a short meditation similar to the standard method.

I used the techniques of remote viewing to scan the outside of the woman's body. I saw that she was blond, a little plump, and that she had a smile on her face. I continued scanning her physical body and was quite unexpectedly drawn to her abdomen. I saw that it was distended, but I didn't sense any wrongness in its vibration. When I projected my consciousness inside her abdomen, to my surprise I saw a basketball. I was shocked since I had never encountered anything like it before. My first thought was that she had a tumor, but with a tumor that size, why would she be smiling? I finally recognized that the woman wasn't sick at all; she was pregnant. From then on, basketballs have become my symbol for pregnancy.

Over the years, I've developed other symbols. Varicose veins always look like strings, anemia looks like diluted blood, arthritis looks like snowflakes resting on bones, and ulcers are volcanoes erupting. Your symbols may differ. With experience you will discover their meanings and will be able to use them effectively in assessment and healing.

## Summary

In this chapter, you learned the techniques of remote viewing. Then you learned to use remote viewing to assess disease in a person's body and subtle field. The case reading I included in this chapter illustrates one way to gain useful experience. You can use case readings with your friends, family, and colleagues.

In the next chapter, you will learn how to increase your healing power by performing yogic breathing. Yogic breathing will enhance and balance the flow of healing energy through your subtle field and physical body. After that, you will learn the techniques of prana healing. Prana healing will enable you to use the vast amount of prana you have in your subtle field to perform healing. You will also learn to perform absentee healing by creating a prana bandage. And you will learn to use prana to recharge your subtle energy field—something a spiritual healer must do on a regular basis.

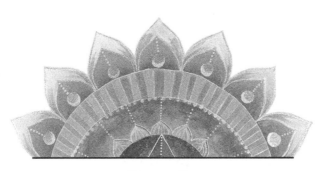

## Part 2

# Self-Healing,
# Absentee Healing,
# and Laying On of Hands

# Chapter 4
# Prana Healing

*Prana* in Sanskrit means "absolute energy or the vital force." Your subtle energy system is composed of prana, and it is prana that vitalizes all your activities. There are many sources of prana in the physical world and non-physical universe. The earth itself radiates prana, as do all living things. Old growth forests radiate vast amounts of prana into the environment and so does the food we eat, especially if it's natural and hasn't been adulterated by excessive processing.

The masters of yoga and tantra recognized that prana was essential for well-being and spiritual development. They learned after careful study that prana flows into a person's field with each breath they take and that resource fields provide people with vast amounts of prana when they are functioning healthfully.

## Pranayama

Prana was so important to the ancient masters of yoga and tantra that they developed pranayama, the science of breath control. In the Bhagavad Gita, we learn that if a yogi becomes a master of pranayama *"he can become one with Brahma ... becoming a co-creator in the All's continuing creation. Using the vital force along with his unconscious mind, he can renew what is neglected and heal what is diseased. His mastery enables him to transmute anything he wants…from state to state; degree to degree; condition to condition…"* [12]

Prana is likened to fire in the Kathopanisad:

> *"Listen, O Naciteka, listen with all attention.*
> *I have the knowledge of fire*
> *which leads the way to immortality.*
> *It is indeed the path to heaven,*
> *this fire—this energy.*
> *It is the support of all creation,*
> *and it is rooted deep within the cave of heart*
> *(the mystery of life)."* [13]

When a healer becomes a master of pranayama, he or she can use the "absolute energy" to renew, to create, and, most importantly, to heal. It's the breath that carries prana in its most concentrated form through a person's physical body and subtle field of energy and consciousness.

## Natural Breathing

The breath is responsible for more than just bringing oxygen into the body. It largely determines a person's state of health by determining the quantity and quality of prana that flows into the person's physical body and subtle fields from the natural environment.

This means that to stay healthy a person must breathe properly. When the breath is not complete, when it's shallow, when a person breathes through the mouth or unconsciously holds their breath between inhalation and exhalation, he or she will weaken the muscles of the diaphragm. Through disuse this disrupts the functions of the lower third the lungs. But more importantly, he or she will disrupt

---

12. Swami, *The Geeta, The Gospel of the Lord Shri Krishna*, 73.

13. Chitrita Devi, *Upanishads for All* (Ram Nagar, New Delhi, India: S. Chand & Co. Ltd., 1973), Kathopanisad 14, 40.

the free flow of prana and the nourishment it brings to the physical body and subtle fields.

## The Yogic Breath

In yoga, there is a technique that will help you remember to breathe properly. This technique is called the *yogic breath*.

The yogic breath is a synthesis of the three basic breaths. The first part is the abdominal breath. In the abdominal breath, you inhale while the abdomen expands and is stretched downward. The second part is the mid breath. In the mid breath, the air that has filled the abdomen is allowed to expand so that it fills the chest cavity. To make room, the rib cage expands and the shoulders lift. The third part is the nasal breath. In the nasal breath, the air that has filled the abdomen and chest is allowed to continue upward until it fills the nasal passages and head.

In complete yogic breathing, not only do you bring more oxygen into your physical body, you stimulate the chakras by bringing prana down through the abdomen and up to the top of the head. Everything vibrates, including prana, and its vibration affects the chakras, keeping them active and functioning harmoniously.

Filling your subtle field with prana and stimulating the chakras will enhance the effect of many of the healing techniques you will learn to perform in this book. So, I encourage you to practice the exercise described below regularly. You will find it very beneficial.

---

### Exercise: Yogic Breathing

To begin yogic breathing, sit in a comfortable position with your back straight and your legs flat on the floor. Once you're sitting comfortably, place your right hand on your abdomen just below the solar plexus. Then close your eyes and inhale through your nose, filling your lower lungs with air. With your hand on your abdomen, you will feel the muscles of your diaphragm stretch as your stomach becomes slightly extended. Continue breathing inward, feeling the air fill the middle and upper part of your lungs. Your shoulders will lift and the muscles of the rib cage will stretch as the lungs expand.

During the mid breath, some people feel pain in the upper back between the shoulder blades. Muscles that have contracted and have become stiff over the years are causing the pain. Don't let a little discomfort discourage you; press on. In a few days, the discomfort will disappear and your muscles will return to their normal state of elasticity.

After air has filled your lungs, let it continue to rise, filling your nasal passages and head, giving you a light, pleasant sensation. When you exhale, reverse the process, letting the nasal passages empty first and then the upper, mid, and finally the lower lungs. Your shoulders will naturally drop and the diaphragm will then return to its normal position.

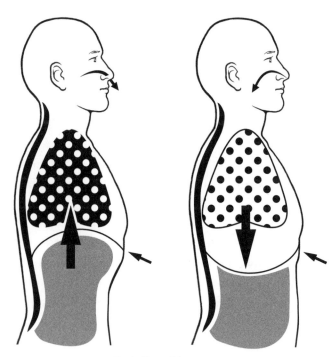

*Yogic Breathing*

Without separation between inhalation and exhalation, continue breathing the same way for ten minutes. Then count from one to five, open your eyes, and bring yourself out of the exercise.

During the first week, practice the exercise for ten minutes. Then increase your practice session to fifteen minutes. If you have a regimen of energy work that you practice regularly, include yogic breathing. Use it to relax before your meditations and before you perform healing. It's an essential element of most of the exercises you will learn to perform in this book.

A NOTE OF WARNING: be sure that you are gentle with yourself! Don't fall victim to watching yourself and your breathing all the time. Don't become obsessive about it because you will simply undermine yourself in other areas, and instead of liberating yourself, you will restrict yourself even more.

## The Fluid Breath

There is a variation of the yogic breath, which I have found useful. It is identical to the previous exercise, except that during inhalation, you imagine a liquid vitality flowing in with the breath. This, of course, is prana, which you see in your visualization as a liquid, or even better, a fluid that is bursting with light and energy. On each inhalation, imagine that this fluid is flowing into your nasal passages, sinuses, bronchial passages, and lungs. On each exhalation, imagine that the fluid is radiating throughout your body, recharging the organs, tissues, cells, and even the molecules themselves. This variation has the added effect of reprogramming your mind and the centers of consciousness throughout your body, including the nuclei of the cells. By visualizing your body being revitalized, even on the cellular level, you create that reality on the mental plane, and then, through transmutation, your cells will be reenergized.

Once you begin practicing the three-part yogic breath, you should soon see positive results. Your vitality will increase and you will be less prone to anxiety and depression. What's more, the nervous chatter and morbid thoughts that accompany those feelings will gradually disappear.

In the next exercise, called the *joint flexibility exercise*, you will use the prana that accompanies your breath to enhance the flexibility of your joints. By doing that, you will enhance the flow of healing energy throughout your physical body and subtle field.

---

## Exercise: Joint Flexibility

You may not realize it, but the prana that continually radiates through your joints provides your body parts with healing energy needed to integrate their functions with the rest of your body and subtle field. Joints that have been denied prana and have contracted are easy to recognize. They can become overly sensitive, numb, or inflexible. In more extreme cases, they can begin to hurt.

The joint flexibility exercise has been designed specifically to overcome the problems associated with inflexibility. By practicing the exercise regularly, you will enhance the flow of prana through your joints that in turn will shrink the blockages that support disease.

To begin the exercise, find a comfortable position with your back straight. Then close your eyes and breathe yogically for two to three minutes. Once you're relaxed, count from five to one and then from ten to one. Then use the standard method to relax your muscles and to center yourself in your subtle field of energy and consciousness.

After you've completed the standard method, focus your mental attention on the vertebrae that connect your neck to your head. Then inhale deeply through the nose, and as you exhale through your nose fill the vertebrae with prana. Repeat the process twice while you remind yourself to let go of any inauthentic desires or emotions, such as jealousy or envy, that may have restricted the free flow of prana through your neck, throat, and shoulders.

Next, bring your attention to your shoulders and the bones, tendons, and muscles that connect them to your arms. Exhale prana through your nose into each shoulder joint twice while you remind yourself to let go of any inauthentic desires or emotions that restricted the free flow of healing energy through them. When you're finished, shake your shoulders loose to let go of any residual heaviness. Then repeat the process with the right and left elbows.

The rib cage is an important area of your body. You will bring prana into your rib cage by exhaling into it. Repeat the process twice while you remind yourself to let go of any beliefs that restrict the free flow of prana through it.

Bring your mental attention to your hips and abdomen next. Place one hand on your lower abdomen and your other hand on your lower back. Stand up and begin to move your hips. With your hands in this position, you will experience the forward, backward, right, and left movements of your hips and pelvis. Then bring prana into your hips and abdomen by exhaling into them twice while you remind yourself to let go of any beliefs that have restricted the free flow of healing energy.

After working on your hips, bring your mental attention to your knees. Try different ways to move them. Then bring prana into your left knee by exhaling into it twice while you remind yourself to let go of any beliefs that have restricted the free flow of healing energy through it. Repeat the same process with your right knee, ankles, toes, wrists, and fingers.

Take about five minutes to fill your remaining joints with prana. Then bring your mental attention to your spine. Make snakelike movements by undulating from top to bottom. Then bring prana into your spine by exhaling into the vertebrae. Repeat the process twice while you remind yourself to let go of any restrictive beliefs. By the time you're done, you'll feel the enhanced flow of healing energy radiating up your back from the base of your spine to the top of your head. Take two to three minutes to enjoy it.

After you've isolated your joints and filled them with healing energy, you are ready to combine your joints and body parts together. Begin by bringing your mental attention to your toes, feet, ankles, and knees. Then continue with your knees and hips moving upward with your mental attention until you feel the enhanced flow of healing energy radiating through your entire physical body. Take a few minutes to enjoy the shift. Then count from one to five and open your eyes.

By the time you've finished the joint flexibility exercise, you should feel more flexible and balanced. You should also feel more healing energy radiating through your physical body, particularly through the body parts that weren't getting the nourishment they needed.

---

## Exercise: Self-Healing with the Prana Bandage

Prana can be used for more than restoring flexibility. It can be used to create a prana bandage. A prana bandage can be used in both self-healing and absentee healing to heal an ailment created by a buildup of distorted energy. In the following exercise, you will use a prana bandage to heal yourself. The process will take five days. After five days, you can repeat the process again if the healing is incomplete.

**Day 1:** To begin, choose a chronic or acute problem in your physical body that you wish to heal. Then find a comfortable position with your back straight. Close your eyes and breathe yogically for two to three minutes. Then count backward from five to one and from ten to one.

Use the standard method to relax your muscles and to center yourself in your subtle field of energy and consciousness. Then assert, "*It's my intent to visualize a screen eight feet (2.5 m) in front of me.*" Continue by asserting, "*It's my intent to visualize myself on the screen.*" Once you appear on the screen, assert, "*It's my intent to mentally project myself inside my body standing next to the organ (or tissue) I've chosen to heal."* View this on the screen. Then take a few moments to scan the area.

Once you're satisfied that you've experienced the distorted fields that support the ailment and their physical manifestation, assert, *"It's my intent to surround both the diseased tissue and the distorted fields that support it with a prana bandage."* Continue by asserting, *"It's my intent that the prana bandage heals the ailment on both the physical and subtle levels."* Don't do anything after that. Just remain centered and let the prana bandage do its work. After ten minutes, release the image of yourself and the screen. Then bring yourself out of the meditation by counting from one to five.

**Days 2 to 4:** On days two, three, and four, find a comfortable position with your back straight. Close your eyes and breathe yogically for two to three minutes. Then count backward from five to one and from ten to one. Use the standard method to relax your muscles and to center yourself in your subtle field of energy and consciousness. Then assert, *"It's my intent to visualize a screen eight feet (2.5 m) in front of me."* Continue by asserting, *"It's my intent to visualize myself on the screen."* Then assert, *"It's my intent to replace my old prana bandage with a new one."*

After you've replaced the prana bandage with a new one, assert, *"It's my intent that prana from the prana bandage is being absorbed by the body part I've chosen to heal."* Take ten minutes more to enjoy the process. After ten minutes, release the image of yourself and the screen. Then bring yourself out of the meditation by counting from one to five.

**Day 5:** On day five, find a comfortable position with your back straight. Close your eyes and breathe yogically for two to three minutes. Then count backward from five to one and from ten to one. Use the standard method to relax your muscles and to center yourself in your subtle field of energy and consciousness. Then assert, *"It's my intent to visualize a screen eight feet (2.5 m) in front of me."* Continue by asserting, *"It's my intent to visualize myself on the screen."*

Once you appear on the screen, assert, "*It's my intent to replace my old prana bandage with a new one.*" After you've replaced the prana bandage with a new one, assert, "*It's my intent to fill the body part I've chosen to heal with prana.*" Give the process two to three minutes. Then visualize that the prana that filled the body part and the prana from the prana bandage have become one large field of prana. Take ten minutes more to enjoy the process. Before you finish, visualize that the ailment you chose to heal is completely healed. Then release the image of yourself and the visual screen. To complete the process, count from one to five. Then open your eyes and bring yourself out of the meditation. Repeat as needed.

## Healing Another Person with a Prana Bandage

In the next exercise, you will use your visual screen and a prana bandage to heal another person. Before you begin, however, it's important to take note: whenever you perform remote viewing and/or absentee healing on another person's physical body or subtle energy field, it's essential to get their permission. Although neither remote viewing nor absentee healing when done correctly is an invasive process, there is no guarantee that you won't inadvertently project your own needs or concerns into their subtle field in the form of energy with individual qualities. This can be healed, of course. (To learn more go to chapter 12.) But any intrusion of foreign energy with individual qualities can be disorientating, especially if the client has no idea that their subtle field is being scanned or an absentee healing is being performed. Then there is also the issue of privacy. A person's subtle field is their private space and this should be respected.

In addition to respecting your client's privacy, it's also essential to have the right attitude when working on another person either through remote viewing, absentee healing, or laying on of hands. You must have confidence in yourself and must inspire confidence in your clients. Through affirmations, plant in your client the conviction that he or she will be healed. Encourage your client to persevere even though, at first, there may be no evidence of improvement. I have found in a majority of cases that perceptible improvement often takes a little while. So nurture your client's initial hope until he or she becomes convinced beyond doubt that he or she will be healed. If nourished, the conviction will blossom into faith, and as we know, with faith all things are possible.

---

### Exercise: Absentee Healing with a Prana Bandage

You can use a prana bandage to heal another person once you've gotten their permission, you've agreed on what needs to be healed, and you've explained what you will do during the healing session. It's also important to agree on a time to perform the healing so that the client is alone and relaxed during the process. Once these conditions have been met, you can begin the five-day process.

**Day 1:** On day one, at the agreed upon time, find a comfortable position with your back straight. Close your eyes and breathe yogically for two to three minutes. Then count backward from five to one and from ten to one. Use the standard method to relax your muscles and to center yourself in your subtle field of energy and consciousness. Then assert, "*It's my intent to visualize a screen eight feet (2.5 m) in front of me.*" Continue by asserting, "*It's my intent to visualize* (client's name here) *on the screen.*" Once your client has appeared on the screen, begin to scan his or her body.

Once you're satisfied that you have the information you need, assert, "*It's my intent to mentally project myself inside* (client's name here)*'s body standing next to the* (organ or tissue) *I've chosen to heal.*" Continue to scan the area. Once you're satisfied that you've seen the ailment in the physical body, as well as the size and shape of the energetic fields that support it, assert, "*It's my intent to surround both the diseased tissue and the subtle fields that support it with a prana bandage.*" Then assert, "*It's my intent that the prana bandage heals the ailment on both the physical and subtle levels.*" Don't do anything after that. Just remain centered and let the prana bandage do its work. After ten minutes, release your client and the visual screen. Then recharge yourself.

When you perform an absentee healing, it's essential to recharge yourself afterward since there is always a slight loss of prana from your subtle field. To do that, assert, "*It's my intent that prana from my resource fields radiates through my subtle field and physical body and recharges them both.*" As soon as you feel your subtle field glowing with energy, count from one to five. When you reach the number five, open your eyes. You will feel wide awake, perfectly relaxed, and better than you did before.

**Days 2 to 4:** On days two, three, and four, at the agreed upon time, find a comfortable position with your back straight. Close your eyes and breathe yogically for two to three minutes. Then count backward from five to one and from ten to one. Use the standard method to relax your muscles and to center yourself in your subtle field of energy and consciousness. Then assert, "*It's my intent to visualize a screen eight feet (2.5 m) in front of me.*" Continue by asserting, "*It's my intent to visualize* (client's name here) *on the screen.*" Then assert, "*It's my intent to replace the old prana bandage with a new one.*" After you've replaced the prana bandage with a new one, assert, "*It's my intent that the new prana bandage heals the ailment on both the physical and subtle levels.*" Take ten minutes more to enjoy the process. After ten minutes, release the image of your client and the screen. Then recharge yourself. When you feel your subtle field glowing with energy, count from one to five and bring yourself out of the meditation.

**Day 5:** On day five, at the agreed upon time, find a comfortable position with your back straight. Close your eyes and breathe yogically for two to three minutes. Then count backward from five to one and from ten to one. Use the standard method to relax your muscles and to center yourself in your subtle field of energy and consciousness. Then assert, "*It's my intent to visualize a screen eight feet (2.5 m) in front of me.*"

Continue by asserting, "*It's my intent to visualize* (client's name here) *on the screen.*" Once your client appears on the screen, assert, "*It's my intent to replace the old prana bandage with a new one.*" After you've replaced the prana bandage with a new one, assert, "*It's my intent to fill the body part I've chosen to heal with prana.*" Give the process two to three minutes. Then visualize that the prana that filled the body part and the prana from the prana bandage have become one large field of prana. Take ten minutes to enjoy the process.

After ten minutes, visualize that the diseased tissue is perfectly healthy. Then release the image of your client and the screen. Take the next few minutes to recharge yourself. When you feel your subtle field glowing with energy, count from one to five and bring yourself out of the meditation.

## Summary

In this chapter, you learned to enhance the flow of prana through your subtle field by performing the three-part yogic breath. Then you learned some basic healing methods that can be extremely effective when used regularly. The first was the joint flexibility exercise. The second was the prana bandage, which you can use for self-healing and to heal other people.

In the next chapter, you will take the next step in healing by learning how your auras function and what auric colors and features tell us about health and disease. From there you will learn to perform auric assessment by sensing, feeling, and seeing the aura. After that, you will learn to perform auric healing by filling your auric field with prana.

# Chapter 5

# Auric Healing

Each auric field is composed of an inner cavity that interpenetrates your subtle field and a thin surface boundary that surrounds it. The aura's internal cavity serves as a reservoir of prana that is instrumental in maintaining vitality and good health. The surface boundary separates your subtle field from the external environment and gives your auras their characteristic egg shape.

Each boundary is composed of luminescent fibers that crisscross each other in every conceivable direction. The composition of the surface boundary makes it permeable, which allows distorted energy to pass through it and to be released. This is a slow process that you will learn to enhance through auric healing later in this chapter.

To perform auric healing, the spiritual healer must be able to see, sense, and feel the aura in order to diagnose problems that cause disease. Then he or she must be able to project healing energy stored in the auric fields to his or her client through the eyes and the minor energy centers in the hands. Everyone has minor energy centers scattered throughout their subtle field. And everyone can use the prana radiating through them to perform auric healing.

## Auric Assessment

The auric fields play an important part in assessment, particularly on the energetic level, for two reasons. First, the subtle energy that causes disease is heavier, denser, and moves more erratically than the energy associated with good health. Second, like sunlight, subtle energy can be broken down into specific colors depending on its frequency. Primary colors that are bright and clear indicate good health. Colors that are muddy, dirty, or associated with earth tones (browns, grays, and black) indicate disease.

I've included a short description of the colors that can appear in the human aura—particularly the etheric aura—along with what each color tells us about the health of a person's body, soul, and spirit.

The etheric aura extends about six inches (15 cm) from the surface of the physical body. By examining the colors and qualities of a client's aura, a healer can tell the nature and severity of the client's disease and determine the kind of energy the client needs to regain health and balance. Then the healer can project the necessary healing energy, in the appropriate color, to the client. This is known as color healing and we will look into it more deeply in the following chapter.

## The Aura's Features

It is generally agreed among researchers that the human aura is more or less egg-shaped and usually follows the contour of the physical body, but this can vary. People with greater vitality will have stronger auric fields, and consequently they will extend farther from the physical body and be more oval in shape.

Also, the composition of the aura varies with each individual. The texture tells us about the character of a person, while the shape and color show us his or her health and emotional condition. A smooth, taut surface indicates personal power, character, and good health. When the surface of the aura is bumpy, flaccid in places, and uneven, it indicates weakness, character flaws, and a lack of balance and well-being. An auric field with colors that have become dirty and muddy and with a surface boundary that has one or more of the defects mentioned above will indicate the presence of physical disease.

## The Auric Colors

There are an astonishing number of colors within the human aura. The following is a list of the most common colors found in the human aura and what they indicate concerning the health of a person's body, soul, and spirit. It's important to note that all the colors of the aura should be bright and clear. The muddier and darker the colors appear, the more likely that a person will have health problems.

## The Red Group

In the human aura, the red group of colors has the lowest visible vibration. It has a dual nature. In its positive form, when it's bright and clear, its aspects are energizing, warming, and exciting. It indicates a solid and secure relationship to the earth. Bright, clear red shows vitality, generosity, and material health. A rosy brightness shows filial affection and the love of home, while red that moves into pink shows happiness and tenderness.

Its negative aspects range from anger and malice to destructiveness and hate. When the red is deep, it indicates passion. When the red is very dark, it indicates selfishness and lack of empathy. Red that has brown in it indicates fear. When the brown darkens and becomes black, it indicates vindictiveness and malice.

When red has a tint of yellow, we see uncontrolled emotions and desires. When we see a light red, it indicates a nervous temperament.

## The Orange Group

Orange, when it's clear and bright, points to strength and vitality as well as sexual passion and enthusiasm. When it becomes reddish, it indicates a person who is self-involved and self-centered.

## The Yellow Group

Yellow is the color of intellect. When it's dull, it indicates intellect, but of a mundane nature. When it becomes brighter, moving into gold, there is an elevation of the intellect and it becomes purified through spirit. Muddy or dirty yellow indicates cunning, greed, and a self-centered, egotistical character.

## The Green Group

Green is the color of balance and harmony. It's the color of the heart. Emerald green, which is clear and bright, indicates an interest or involvement in the healing arts. Light green indicates a peaceful nature and an affinity for the outdoors. In its negative form, when it's muddy and dirty, green can indicate extreme selfishness, deceit, and greed. When it becomes brownish, it indicates jealousy.

## The Blue Group

Blue has always been associated with religious sensitivity and intuitive awareness. In its highest form, blue is associated with inspiration and the higher forms of intellect. It's one of the first colors a healer sees. On the negative side, blue with brown or black in it indicates a fascination with the darker side of spirituality.

## The Violet Group

Violet, which is a combination of red and blue, points to even loftier spiritual ideals and power. Those who have violet in their aura have advanced farthest in their spiritual journey. Violet in the aura acts as an insulator and purifier. It can be observed most often in the auric fields of spiritual masters and adepts. When it shades into lavender, it denotes a high level of spirituality as well as a great deal of vitality. When it shades into lilac, it shows a compassionate and altruistic character.

Violet first appears above the head. As the adept advances, the violet radiates from there until it fills his or her entire aura with its light.

## The Silver Group

Silver pertains to spiritual and physical abundance. Bright silver in the aura can mean spiritual awakening or the accumulation of physical and spiritual wealth. Clear metallic silver is nurturing, intuitive, and indicates a creative mind. When the silver has streaks of gray or it has become muddy, it indicates fear and body image problems. Heavier and denser gray indicates blocked energy and the likelihood of physical disease.

## The Gold Group

Gold pertains to divine strength and worldly wisdom. People with gold in their aura listen to their inner voice and receive a continuous stream of insight to guide them. They remain free of worldly attachments and enjoy the benefits of a blissful life.

## The Brown Group

Brown is a combination of all colors but is not itself a color found in the spectrum. Some researchers connect brown with business and industry, calling it the businessman's color. But normally, it's a color associated with physical disease. Most healers associate brown with negative human characteristics. In its various forms, it indicates stinginess, greed, and a lack of character. Only when it becomes a golden brown does its vibration rise, showing an industrious, organized character and a methodical temperament.

## Black

Black, which is the absence of light, indicates darkness on all levels. When black has filled a person's aura, it indicates the negation of life itself. When streaks of black are seen within an otherwise normal aura, they tend to neutralize the good aspects of what would have been a healthy aura.

## The Gray Group

Gray is also a negative color. It's associated with a dull, conventional character. It also indicates a lack of vitality, depression, and physical disease. Heavy, deep grays indicate fear, confusion, and, in some cases, an unreliable, deceptive character.

## White

Finally, we come to white, which is the synthesis of all colors. When it appears in a person's aura, it indicates balance, harmony, and the capacity for intimacy and union. It's the color of spiritual perfection and is found only in those people who've achieved enlightenment.

# The Etheric Aura

Now that you know what the colors and features in the aura indicate, you're ready to have a direct experience of the etheric aura. The etheric auric is the field that will provide you with the most immediate information about the condition of your subject's body, soul, and spirit. There are three ways that you can experience the aura. You can feel the surface of the aura through your palms, you can see the aura clairvoyantly, and you can see the aura by developing auric vision.

In the following exercise, you will learn to feel the aura with your palms. Afterward, you will learn to use clairvoyance and auric vision to view and diagnose disease in the etheric aura.

---

### Exercise: Stroking the Etheric Aura

Each of you has the capacity to feel the etheric aura and to sense its condition through the palms of your hands. By stroking the surface of your subject's aura with the palm of your hand, you can collect information about the physical health, character, and emotional well-being of your subject. Stroking the surface of the etheric aura is a simple technique. To perform it, you will need a willing subject. Explain to your subject what you will be doing, then follow these simple instructions.

To begin the exercise, have your subject lie down on his or her back. If he or she doesn't meditate or do spiritual exercises, have your subject breathe deeply through the nose with eyes closed for two to three minutes. Since changes can occur in your subject's aura as a result of strong feelings, excitement, or anxiety, having them relaxed is essential for receiving accurate impressions.

As soon as your subject has closed his or her eyes, begin to breathe yogically. Then close your eyes and perform the standard method to relax the muscles of your body and to center yourself in your subtle field of energy and consciousness. Once you're centered, open your eyes, stand up, and place your positive hand (right hand if you're right-handed, left hand if you're left-handed) about a foot (30 cm) above your subject's heart. Bring your mental attention to your palm. Then let your hand descend until you feel a slight resistance, which will make the palm of your hand tingle. The resistance comes from the surface of your subject's etheric aura.

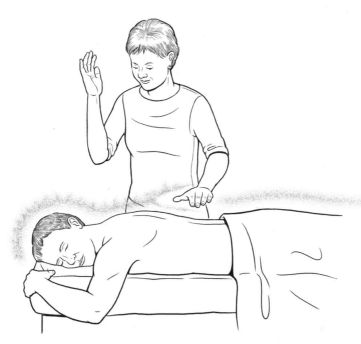

**Stroking the Etheric Aura**

As soon as you feel resistance, begin skimming the surface of your subject's aura. Always keep your palm on the surface. Only in that way will you receive accurate impressions of the aura's strength and texture. If you allow your hand to pass through the surface, you will feel the energy of your own hand as it is reflected off your subject's body. If you get close enough to his or her physical body, you will feel the heat generated by the body and nothing more.

As you skim the surface of your subject's aura, become aware of changes in the aura's energy level. Changes can cause your hand to dip toward your subject's body or to be pushed farther away from it. Sharp changes signify problems in your subject's subtle field. Note differences in temperature. Cold spots and warm spots can also indicate the presence of energetic problems and potential disease.

The aura should be firm, smooth, and a uniform temperature. Whenever these conditions are altered, disease of some sort is the culprit. After you've registered all the impressions from the front, have your subject turn over and continue the process on his or her back. In the beginning, be sure to get feedback. With practice, you will become more sensitive and more confident, and you will recognize the sensations associated with different diseases and conditions.

After you've scanned the surface of your subject's etheric aura and you're satisfied with your findings, remove your hand, sit down again, and take a moment to relax.

If you're already a practitioner or you intend to become one, it would be a good idea to keep a catalogue of your findings. Every disease or ailment gives off a specific vibration, and if you practice auric assessment regularly, you will learn to discern the signature of different ailments in body, soul, and spirit.

---

### Exercise: Auric Viewing

Another method of auric assessment is auric viewing. There are no limitations to this technique. It can be used anytime and anywhere, whether you're with your client or not. It can be used in association with other diagnostic techniques, so it should be developed by anyone who will be working as a spiritual healer.

To view the aura clairvoyantly, begin breathing yogically for two to three minutes. Then use the standard method to relax your muscles and center yourself in your subtle field of energy and consciousness. Once you're centered, assert, "*It's my intent to create my visual screen eight feet (2.5 m) in front of me.*" Continue by asserting, "*It's my intent to visualize* (subject's name here) *on the screen in front of me."* As soon as your subject appears on the screen, look past them until your vision blurs. In a short time, you will see what looks like mist surrounding his or her body. Continue for a short time longer and colors will begin to emerge. As soon as they do, begin using the techniques of remote viewing to scan your subject's etheric aura.

Be attentive to anything that doesn't look or feel right. Problems will stand out and draw your attention. You might be looking at the aura around your subject's head, and suddenly you'll get a sense of wrongness and be drawn to the knee. When that happens, you can be confident that your subject has a problem with his or her knee. If there is a problem with the knee or any other body part, examine the etheric aura surrounding it. Pay attention to the color, texture, and strength.

It's important to note that an experienced healer will combine auric assessment with remote viewing once they've seen one or more defects in the aura around a particular body part. I recommend that you do the same. If you see defects in the etheric aura surrounding one of your client's body parts, project yourself inside his or her physical body and examine the body part in more detail. (For more information on remote viewing, go to chapter 3.)

In serious ailments, such as heart disease, you will probably see negative colors in the aura. But you might not see the connection between various energetic markers in the aura and their physical manifestation unless you use the techniques of remote viewing to project yourself inside your subject's body.

After you've examined the aura clairvoyantly and validated what you've learned by using the techniques of remote viewing, assert, *"It's my intent to project myself back to my original position eight feet (2.5 m) in front of my visual screen."* Release your subject and the screen next. Then recharge yourself. After you've recharged yourself, count from one to five and bring yourself out of the exercise.

# The Aura and Dr. Kilner

The English scientist Walter J. Kilner pioneered scientific research into the human aura. In 1908, Kilner came up with the idea that the aura could be made visible if viewed through a screen coated with a suitable dye. He experimented with Dicyanin, a coal tar derivative, and found it had an extraordinary effect on eyesight.[14] He discovered the coal tar produced a temporary shortsightedness when people gazed through a screen coated with it. When they looked through it, people became more sensitive to radiation from the ultraviolet end of the spectrum. For some reason, this increased sensitivity allowed people to see the etheric aura clearly. Kilner also found that the aura was more visible when light was shaded, and he conducted most of his experiments in semi-darkened rooms. Later he discovered that a black background improved auric vision. Therefore, in many of his subsequent experiments, he placed a subject in a darkened room about ten inches (30 cm) from a dark wall and then examined the person through the Dicyanin screen.

In later years, it was discovered that the screen could be discarded because it was the temporary shortsightedness that made the aura visible. Shortsightedness can be achieved easily by simply looking past an object until the eyes unfocus.

# Seeing the Aura

In the hundred years since Dr. Kilner's pioneering research, it's been discovered that three conditions must be met in order to physically see the etheric aura. First, the observer must be centered in their subtle field of energy and consciousness. This allows the healer to see subtle fields more clearly. Second, the space where viewing takes place must be darkened and a dark background must be behind the person being viewed. Lastly, the observer must allow his eyes to unfocus without straining them.

Clothes can interfere with your ability to see that aura surrounding a person's torso, so in most cases the aura is most readily seen around

---

14. Walter J. Kilner, *Human Aura* (Secaucus, NJ: Citadel Press, 1965).

the head, hands, and feet. In the exercise that follows, you will view the aura around your hands. To do that, you will need a black piece of stiff paper about three feet (90 cm) long and eighteen inches (46 cm) wide.

---

### Exercise: Seeing Your Aura

To see your etheric aura, find a comfortable position with your back straight. Breathe yogically for two to three minutes. Then use the standard method to relax your muscles and to center yourself in your subtle field of energy and consciousness. Take a few moments to enjoy the shift. Then affirm, *"I'm in the perfect condition to see the aura around my hands."* Look past your hands into the paper below them. For best results, your hands should be held three inches (8 cm) above the paper in a horizontal position, palms up, with the fingers pointing toward each other and almost touching. The fingers should be comfortably spread out. Once you've begun to look past your hands and through your fingers, your eyes will unfocus without any difficulty.

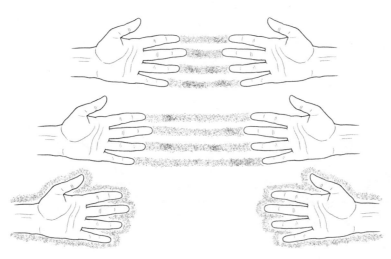

*Auric Vision*

At first, the aura may be faint and difficult to see; it might look something like steam evaporating. But if you continue to pay attention without concentrating, the aura will get brighter. As the brightness grows stronger, colors will begin to emerge. When this happens, slowly spread your hands apart and you will see lines of force connecting your fingers. These lines will connect the corresponding fingers of each hand and will join them together until you've spread the hands six to eight inches (15 to 20 cm) apart. Then the lines will split down the center and you will see the aura surrounding each hand separately.

After you've mastered this technique, it will become progressively easier for you to see the colors around your hands. When you feel confident of your ability, begin examining the auras of your friends and associates. The auras around their heads will be easiest for you to see.

---

## Exercise: Viewing Another Person's Aura

When you want to see another person's aura, use the standard method to relax your muscles and to center yourself in your subtle energy field of energy and consciousness. Make sure that there is a clear background behind the person being viewed. Black or white will work best. Then unfocus your eyes and look past your subject into the clear background. The aura around the head will emerge first as a mist, then in colors, with the dark colors emerging first, followed by the lighter colors. The aura will resemble the halos that you've seen in portraits of saints. Once you've mastered the technique, the auric colors will become as bright or even brighter than the colors you see in the physical world.

Most healers I know use at least one of the techniques you learned in this chapter, along with remote viewing, for assessment. Practice them all and use the combination that works best for you.

Before we move on to auric healing, it's important to re-member that your body is an instrument that will register dis-comforts from another person's body when you attune yourself to his or her vibration. So, expect to feel unusual sensations in your own body when you practice auric assessment. These dis-comforts are temporary. They're a form of psychic communi-cation that you should learn to use along with remote viewing and auric assessment to diagnose disease.

## Auric Healing

Now that you've learned the three techniques of auric assessment, you're ready to perform auric healing by filling your etheric aura with prana. By filling your etheric aura with prana, you will enhance the pressure within it. Enhancing the pressure will help the aura retain its integrity, especially when it comes into contact with fields of distort-ed energy that could potentially disrupt it. Filling your etheric aura with prana will also enhance your vitality, self-confidence, and overall health by replacing distorted fields of energy with healing energy.

---

### Exercise: Filling the Etheric Aura with Prana

To begin the exercise, find a comfortable position with your back straight. Then close your eyes and breathe yogically for two to three minutes. Continue by counting backward from five to one and from ten to one. Use the standard method to relax your muscles and to center yourself in your subtle field of energy and consciousness. Then assert, "*It's my intent to center myself in my subtle field on the etheric level.*" Continue by asserting, "*It's my intent to turn my organs of perception inward in my subtle field on the etheric level.*" Take a few moments to enjoy the process. Then assert, "*It's my intent to fill my etheric aura with prana.*" Take fif-teen minutes to experience the shift. Then bring yourself out of the exercise by counting from one to five. When you reach the number five, open your eyes. You will feel wide awake, perfectly relaxed, and better than you did before. Repeat as needed.

In the exercise you just performed, you filled your etheric aura with prana. To perform the same exercise on the other dimensions of your body, soul, and spirit, simply choose a different auric field to work on. On the material level, you can work on the lower physical-material aura, the upper physical-material aura, the lower physical aura, upper physical aura, lower etheric aura, and upper etheric aura.

On the level of soul, you can work on the aura surrounding the second chakra, third chakra, fourth chakra, and fifth chakra. On the level of spirit, you can work on the aura surrounding your sixth and seventh chakras.

Before we move on, it's important to remember that every time you fill an auric field with prana, you will strengthen your subtle field, weaken attachments that block you, and enhance your physical health and well-being.

## Summary

In this chapter, you learned to use your auric fields as a diagnostic tool. With practice, auric assessment will become one of your most valuable resources. You also learned to heal your auric fields by filling them with prana. As a way of maintaining wellness and enhancing your level of vitality, this technique is unsurpassed.

In the following chapter, you will learn to use your intent and mental attention in combination with your eyes and the minor energy centers in your hands to perform advanced auric healing on yourself and other people.

# Chapter 6
# Advanced Auric Healing

In advanced auric healing, you will project prana stored in your auric fields to the diseased area of your client's body through your eyes and palms. We will begin our study by looking at the eyes and how they can be used in advanced auric healing. Then we will look at the palms and the energy centers contained within them.

Although the eyes are not structurally part of your subtle field, spiritual healers have known for centuries that they have the power to radiate healing energy. In the sixth chapter of Matthew, we are told that *"the light of the body is in the eye..."*[15] In fact, a strong, steady gaze fueled by prana can be used to enhance your healing power and to heal the sick. Using your eyes in this way is called gazing. When you gaze at someone, you will be connecting your eyes to healing energy stored in your etheric aura. Then you will project that energy through your eyes to the part of your client's body that needs it.

You can use gazing in combination with other techniques of auric healing in absentee healing and later when you learn to perform laying on of hands. It's important to note that gazing does not mean staring. When I use gazing, I don't concentrate—rather I focus my mental attention on the body part I've chosen to heal and then enjoy the process as healing energy radiates from my etheric aura, through my eyes, into the diseased tissue.

---

15. Matt. 6:22 (KJV).

## Exercise: Strengthening Your Gaze

Before you can use your eyes to radiate healing energy, you must first strengthen your gaze and learn to focus it. To do that, you will need a large mirror. Place the mirror about three feet (1 m) in front of you so that you can see your whole face clearly.

When you're ready to begin, sit in front of the mirror with your back straight. Then close your eyes and breathe yogically for two to three minutes. Continue by counting from five to one, then from ten to one. Use the standard method to relax the muscles and center yourself in your subtle field of energy and consciousness. Then assert, "*It's my intent to center myself in my subtle field.*" Once you're centered, open your eyes (keep them slightly unfocused) and make eye contact with the image of yourself in the mirror. Once you've made contact, assert, "*It's my intent to turn my organs of perception inward on the level of my subtle field.*" Take two to three minutes to enjoy the shift. Then assert, "*It's my intent to radiate prana through my eyes to the image of myself in the mirror.*" Don't do anything after that. Don't try to understand what's happening or to give the prana an extra push. Just enjoy the process for ten more minutes while you continue to make eye contact. After ten minutes, count from one to five. Then release eye contact and bring yourself out of the exercise. Repeat every day for five days or until you feel confident that you can use gazing as part of your healing sessions.

Once you're confident that you can radiate prana through your eyes without disruption, you can substitute your visual screen for the mirror and practice auric healing on yourself and/or another person.

## Exercise: Auric Healing by Gazing

In the following exercise, you will use your eyes to perform an auric healing on yourself. Before you begin, choose an ailment you wish to heal. Then find a comfortable position with your back straight. Close your eyes and breathe yogically next. Then count from five to one and from ten to one. Use the standard method to relax the muscles and to center yourself in your subtle field of energy and consciousness.

Once you're centered, assert, *"It's my intent to create a visual screen eight feet (2.5 m) in front of me."* Then assert, *"It's my intent to visualize an image of myself on the screen."* As soon as you see the image of yourself appear, assert, *"It's my intent to fill my etheric aura with prana."* Once you feel your etheric aura glowing with energy, begin gazing at the body part you've chosen to heal. Then assert, *"It's my intent to radiate prana from my etheric aura through my eyes and into the body part I've chosen to heal."* Continue to gaze at the body part for five minutes. At the end of the process, visualize that the body part is perfectly healthy and glowing with energy. Then release the energy you've been projecting through your eyes. Release the image of yourself and the visual screen next. Then count from one to five and bring yourself out of the healing meditation. Repeat as needed.

## Auric Healing with the Hands

In addition to gazing, you can perform auric healing by projecting prana through the minor energy centers in your hands. The minor energy centers in your hands are part of your subtle energy system and work in conjunction with your resource fields, chakras, meridians, and auric fields. However, in contrast to these other organs that have fixed structures, the minor energy centers in your hands are created by the interaction of two ruling meridians, which means they function exclusively as centers of activity.

The energy centers in your hands have several functions that enhance your ability to express yourself, participate in worldly activities, and perform auric healing. They augment your ability to manifest all your functions of mind including will, desire, creativity, and love. And they allow you to share healing energy with people who need it.

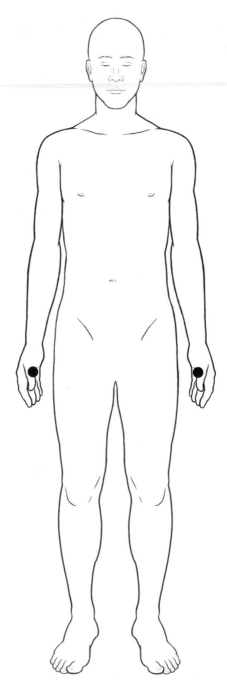

*The Minor Energy Centers in the Hands*

In the following exercise, you will learn to enhance the functions of the energy centers in your hands by increasing the flow of prana through the meridians that terminate in your palms. They're known as Yang Yu and Yin Yu meridians. Before you do that, however, it will be useful to learn more about how your meridians function and promote the flow of healing energy.

## Meridians

Meridians are channels that transmit healing energy throughout your subtle field and physical body. They keep the human energy system in balance and they help to maintain its integrity by connecting the chakras to each other and to the minor energy centers scattered throughout the subtle field.

Although functionally the meridians correspond to the veins and arteries of the circulatory system, structurally they closely resemble currents of water and/or air found in Earth's oceans and atmosphere. As a result, their size, shape, and carrying capacity can change depending on the quantity of energy they carry, the condition of the first and seventh chakras, the minor energy centers in the hands and feet, and variations in pressure exerted by fields of distorted energy in their immediate environment. Their unique structure makes it possible for them to rapidly increase or decrease in size and carrying capacity. They even shift position, if necessary, as the quality and quantity of prana flowing through them changes.

## Function of the Meridians

Individually and collectively, meridians have four important functions:

1. They connect the organs of the subtle energy system to one another.
2. They regulate pressure within the subtle field. They do this by expanding and contracting as the quantity of prana changes and by shifting prana (as needed) from one part of the human energy system to another.

3. The meridians release toxins that have accumulated within energetic vehicles. Toxic energy within an energetic vehicle will be absorbed into the system of meridians, which will transfer the toxins to the appropriate chakra. From the chakra, the toxins will be expelled into the appropriate auric field. Globules of toxic energy will then make their way to the auric surface and over time will be released into the external environment.

4. In their final function, meridians allow prana that is ready to make the quantum jump to be transmitted from the etheric level to the physical body. The energy made available in this way will be used to charge the nerves and to integrate the functions of the physical body with their corresponding energetic vehicles in the subtle field. So all energetic vehicles as well as the physical body will react synchronistically to environmental stimulus.

### The Ruling Meridians

According to ancient texts, there are ten ruling meridians. When it comes to the minor energy centers in the hands, the meridians that are most important are the Yang Yu and Yin Yu. They form the minor energy centers in the palms.

**The Yang Yu:** The (two) Yang Yu meridians are the masculine arm channels located in both arms. They link the shoulders with the centers in the palms, after passing through the middle fingers.

**The Yin Yu:** The Yin Yu meridians are feminine arm channels that link the centers in the palms with the chest. They travel along the insides of each arm.

In the next exercise, you will enhance the function of the minor energy centers in the hands by stimulating the flow of prana through the Yang Yu and Yin Yu meridians, first on the right side of your body and then on the left. As the flow of prana through each circuit increases, your minor energy centers in your hands will become more active and you will receive valuable information about their condition.

## Exercise: The Yin Yu and Yang Yu Meditation

To begin the Yin Yu and Yang Yu meditation, find a comfortable position with your back straight. Then breathe yogically for two to three minutes. Count backward from five to one, then from ten to one. Then use the standard method to relax your muscles and center yourself in your subtle field of energy and consciousness.

Take a few moments to enjoy the shift. Then assert, "*It's my intent to project my mental attention to the upper end of the Yang Yu meridian on the right side of my body.*" If there are no obstructions, the moment your mental attention reaches the Yang Yu the prana flowing through the meridian will carry it down the meridian to its terminus in the palm of the hand. As soon as your mental attention reaches the terminus, shift your mental attention about an inch (2.5 cm) diagonally down toward the base of your hand using the prana that enters with each inhalation. This is the access point of the Yin Yu meridian (in the right palm). If there are no obstructions, the moment you locate the meridian, your mental attention will be carried up the inside of your arm (by the prana flowing through the meridian) to its terminus on the right side of your chest. Once the circuit has been completed, release your mental attention. Remain centered in your subtle field and enjoy the enhanced flow of prana in your palm center and the Yin Yu and Yang Yu meridians.

When you're ready to proceed to the second part of this exercise, assert, "*It's my intent to project my mental attention to the access point of the left Yang Yu meridian.*" If there are no obstructions, the moment you locate the access point your mental attention will be carried down to the meridian's terminus in the palm of the left hand. Move your attention one inch (2.5 cm) diagonally down the palm, at a forty-five-degree angle away from your thumb. There you'll find the access point of the Yin Yu meridian. Let the prana flowing through the meridian carry your mental attention to the terminus in the chest. Then release your mental attention and take fifteen minutes to en-joy the effects of the exercise. After fifteen minutes, count from one to five. When you reach the number five, open your eyes. You will feel wide awake, perfectly relaxed, and better than you did before. Practice the exercise regularly and you will enhance your ability to perform auric healing as well as to manifest your creativity and soul urge in the world.

---

## Exercise: Auric Healing with Your Hands

In the next exercise, you will choose a body part you wish to heal. Then you will fill your etheric aura with prana. After that, you will visualize your own image on the visual screen. Once the image appears, you will project healing energy (from your etheric aura) through the energy centers in your palms to the body part (on the screen) you've chosen to heal.

To begin, find a comfortable position with your back straight. Then close your eyes and breathe yogically for two to three min-utes. Continue by counting from five to one, then from ten to one. Use the standard method to relax your muscles and to cen-ter yourself in your subtle field of energy and consciousness.

Once you're centered, assert, "*It's my intent to fill my etheric aura with prana.*" Take a few moments to enjoy the shift. Then assert, "*It's my intent to create a visual screen eight feet (2.5 m) in front of me.*" Continue by asserting, "*It's my intent to visualize an image of myself on the screen.*" As soon as the image of your-self appears, bring your palms up so that they face the image on the screen. Then assert, "*It's my intent to radiate prana from my etheric aura through my minor energy centers in my palms to the part of my body I've chosen to heal.*" Visualize the energy flowing through your hands into the body part as luminous rays. Continue to radiate the energy for ten minutes. After ten minutes, visualize that the body part is perfectly healthy. Then release the rays of energy from your hands, the image of your-self on the screen, and the visual screen. Count from one to five next. Then open your eyes and bring yourself out of the healing meditation. Repeat as needed.

---

### Exercise: The Complete Auric Healing

You can use the two techniques of auric healing you just learned to perform absentee healing. First, get the person's permission, agree on a time for the healing, and explain what you will doing during the healing session. Before you begin the session, decide what ailment you will be treating.

When you are ready to begin, find a comfortable position with your back straight. Close your eyes and breathe yogically for two to three minutes. Then count from five to one, then from ten to one. Use the standard method to relax your muscles and to center yourself in your subtle field of energy and consciousness.

Once you're centered, assert, "*It's my intent to fill my etheric aura with prana.*" Once you feel your etheric aura glowing with energy, assert, "*It's my intent to create a visual screen eight feet (2.5 m) in front of me.*" Then assert, "*It's my intent to visualize an image of* (client's name here) *on the screen.*" As soon as your client appears, scan the area of their body and the auric field above it. Once you've validated the assessment, assert, "*It's my intent to radiate prana from my etheric aura through my eyes to the part of my client's body I've chosen to heal.*" Continue to gaze for five minutes. Then assert, "*It's my intent to mentally project myself inside my client's body next to the diseased tissue I've chosen to heal.*" Put one hand on one side of the diseased tissue and the other hand opposite it. Then assert, "*It's my intent to radiate healing energy from my etheric aura through the minor energy centers in my palms to the body part I've chosen to heal.*" Continue the healing for ten minutes. Feel your client absorbing the healing energy you're projecting through your palms into the diseased tissue.

After ten minutes, visualize that the diseased tissue is perfectly healthy and glowing with prana. Then mentally project yourself back to your seat in front of the screen. Release your client and the screen next. Then take a few moments to recharge yourself. When you feel your subtle field glowing with energy, count from one to five and bring yourself out of the healing session. Repeat as needed.

## Summary

In this chapter, you learned to strengthen your gaze. Then you learned to perform auric healing by gazing and by projecting healing energy through the minor energy centers in your palms. In the final exercise of this chapter, you combined the techniques you learned to perform a complete auric healing.

In the next chapter, you will learn the basics of chakra healing. You will learn how to activate your chakras and center yourself in your chakra fields. Once you've learned to center yourself in a chakra field, you will be ready to perform an exercise called chakra balancing. Chakra balancing will enable you to enhance and balance the flow of prana through your seven traditional chakras.

# Chapter 7
# Chakra Healing

In order to use your chakras effectively as healing tools, you must first learn how they interact with your subtle field and the other organs of your subtle energy system, particularly the meridians and auric fields. That's because in the same way that problems can occur in modern rail and air terminals when traffic becomes blocked, problems can occur in your subtle field and physical body when the chakras become blocked. These problems, which originate in higher dimensional fields, create fertile ground for the development of disease in your body, soul, and spirit.

In order to rectify problems in the chakras and prevent the development of disease, I've developed simple exercises that will activate your chakras and balance their activity with the rest of your subtle field.

## The Subtle Field

Chakras are energetic vortices contained within your subtle field. Your subtle field is a field of consciousness and subtle energy with universal qualities (prana) that interpenetrates your physical body. It contains bodies of consciousness and two types of energetic vehicles—energy bodies and sheaths. In addition to bodies of consciousness and energetic vehicles, your subtle field contains resource fields and a subtle energy system. Resource fields provide the energy and consciousness your vehicles of energy and your subtle energy system need to function healthfully.

Your subtle energy system includes the chakras and chakra fields, meridians, auras, and minor energy centers scattered through your subtle field. It's through your subtle energy system that prana is transmitted and transmuted into the exact frequencies necessary for you to participate successfully in all the normal activities of life.

## The Chakras

The word *chakra* comes from Sanskrit and means "wheel." There are two distinct parts of a chakra—the chakra gate and the chakra field. For people with the ability to see subtle energy fields, a chakra gate will look like a brightly colored disk that spins rapidly at the end of what looks like a long axle or stalk. The wheel portion of the chakra gate is about three inches (8 cm) in diameter and perpetually moves or spins around a central axis. Emerging from the center of the disk are what appear to be spokes.

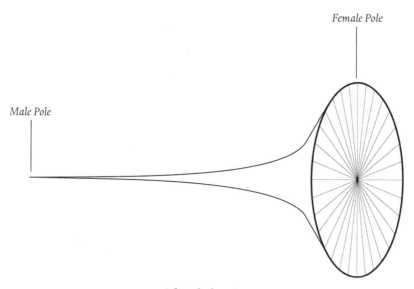

*The Chakra Gate*

The main function of the chakra gate is to provide the subtle field and physical body with prana. Although chakra gates have additional functions, the principle part of a chakra is the vast reservoir of prana, which we call the chakra field. The chakra field is connected to the chakra gate. And the healthier the chakra field, the more prana will be distributed by the chakra gate to your subtle field and physical body.

## Functions of the Chakras

The chakra gates and chakra fields are primarily responsible for regulating energetic activities in the non-physical universe. These activities include many interactions that people mistakenly believe take place exclusively on the physical plane. Empathy, motivation, and enthusiasm, as well as human love and intimacy, are examples of energetic interactions regulated by the chakras and chakra fields.

Chakra gates and their fields are able to perform these essential functions because they provide your subtle energy system and physical body with prana, and they transmute prana from one pitch (or frequency) to another whenever an energy body, sheath, or your physical body is in an energy-deficient condition. In addition, they link all human beings to Universal Consciousness.

Chakras also help balance the forces of polarity and gender in your energy field by permitting prana to move through your subtle energy system. It moves in four general directions—up the back, down the front, forward from the back to the front, and backward from the front to the back.

Maintaining a healthy balance between the forces of polarity and gender by distributing prana from one part of your subtle energy system to another will empower you and enhance your ability to express yourself fully.

## The Thirteen Chakras in Body Space

There are 146 chakras within the human energy system. The thirteen most important chakras are located within your body space. These include the seven traditional chakras located along the spine and in the head, two etheric chakras, two physical chakras, and two physical-material chakras.

Below is a short list of the individual activities regulated by the thirteen chakras in body space and the functions of spirit, soul, and body they regulate.

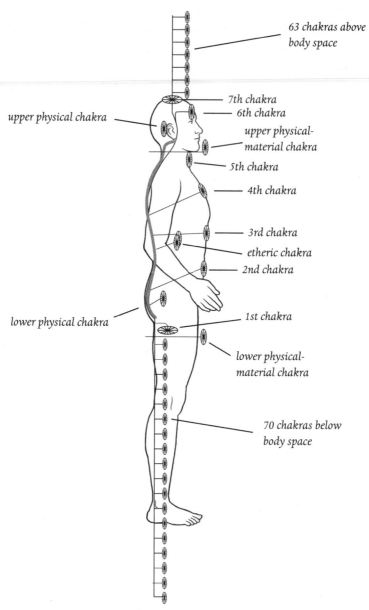

*63 chakras above body space*

*7th chakra*
*6th chakra*

*upper physical chakra*

*upper physical-material chakra*

*5th chakra*

*4th chakra*

*3rd chakra*

*etheric chakra*

*2nd chakra*

*lower physical chakra*

*1st chakra*

*lower physical-material chakra*

*70 chakras below body space*

**Chakras in Body Space**

**First Chakra:** The first or root chakra is located at the base of the spine and is fiery orange-red when active. It is a channel for subtle energies entering the earth plane. When it's functioning properly, a person feels a deep personal attachment to the earth. Security, self-confidence, and body image are additional qualities associated with the first chakra. If the chakra is blocked, your relationship to the earth will be disrupted and so will your relationship to your physical body.

**Second Chakra:** The second chakra is located four finger widths below the naval. It corresponds to the sun, and, when it's active, it radiates prana in the orange spectrum. It regulates vitality, gender identity (masculinity or femininity), creativity, and physical joy. If the chakra is blocked, you will experience anger and a loss of physical vitality.

**Third Chakra:** The third chakra is the solar plexus center. It's through the third chakra that people feel connected to the physical and etheric world. For the average person, it's the seat of the personality. This chakra is associated with the color yellow. It regulates belonging, contentment, intimacy, friendship, status, and psychic well-being. If the chakra is blocked, you will experience fear as well as a lack of trust in yourself and in other people.

**Fourth Chakra:** The fourth chakra is the heart center. It emerges from the spine and extends to the center of the breastbone. When active, it glows with a bright green color. It's the source of light and love. The heart chakra regulates self-awareness and personal rights (this includes the right to control your physical body, to express your feelings and emotions, and to share your knowledge with other people). If the chakra is blocked, you will experience pain as well as a longing for a deeper connection to the world of spirit.

**Fifth Chakra:** The fifth chakra is known as the throat chakra. To the trained clairvoyant, it appears silvery blue, oftentimes with a hint of green. The chakra gate emerges from the back of the neck, just below your medulla oblongata, and reaches downward toward the front of the throat just below the Adam's apple. It regulates all forms of human expression as well as enjoyment, perseverance, and personal integrity. If the chakra is blocked, so is your experience of unconditional joy and your ability to express yourself freely.

**Sixth Chakra:** The sixth chakra is alternately called the brow chakra or the third eye. It's located directly between and slightly above the eyebrows. It radiates a deep blue hue when it's functioning healthfully. The sixth chakra is directly linked to seeing, not only in the physical sense but in the mystical sense of seeing into the higher planes. Awareness, memory, intuition, reasoning, and deductive thought, as well as clairvoyance and the other paranormal forms of knowing, are additional qualities regulated by the chakra. If the chakra is blocked, you will experience a disruption in inductive and deductive reasoning, memory, and intuition.

**Seventh Chakra:** The seventh chakra is known as the crown chakra. When active, it's the most vibrant of the seven traditional chakras. Although it appears to vibrate in a host of colors, to the trained eye it's predominantly violet. The crown chakra emerges from a point one inch (2 cm) above the pituitary gland and extends to the top of the head. It's called the "thousand-petaled lotus" in Hindu scripture. According to the Hindus, it's associated with transcendental consciousness. If the chakra is blocked, your experience of self-realization and transcendent relationship will also be blocked.

**Etheric Chakras:** These chakras regulate feelings. There are hundreds of authentic feelings that emerge from the etheric chakras. They range from comfort and satisfaction to fatigue and enthusiasm. If the chakras are blocked, your access to feelings and your ability to express them will be blocked.

**Physical Chakras:** These chakras are responsible for regulating physical pleasure, particularly sexual pleasure. When the physical chakras are blocked, you will feel locked outside of yourself on the physical level, with a corresponding loss of passion and sensitivity to other people.

**Physical-Material Chakras:** These chakras are responsible for grounding you in the physical-material world. Being grounded allows you to experience your physical body and your physical environment without disruption. When the physical-material chakras are blocked, strength and stamina will be disrupted. So will the production of pleasure-producing compounds in the brain.

## Exercises: Sensing the Chakras in Body Space

In my work, I've found that even when people have learned something about the structure and function of the chakras, they're unable to sense them. This is unfortunate because there are simple ways to sense the chakras. One way is to use the power of running water to stimulate them.

This is easy to do in the shower. Simply direct the stream of water from the shower head to the front of your first chakra gate, which extends from the base of your spine to a point three inches (8 cm) below it. Continue until you feel a vibration emerging from the point where the chakra gate is located. Take a moment to enjoy the resonance, then move the shower head to the second chakra gate, which is four finger widths below the navel. After a few moments, you will feel the unique vibration of the second chakra. Continue to use the water emerging from the nozzle to stimulate your third through seventh chakras, and your etheric, physical, and physical-material chakras. You can see the position of the chakras by consulting the *Chakras in Body Space* figure on page 88.

Once you've stimulated all thirteen chakras, take about ten minutes to enjoy their enhanced resonance, which will continue even after you've finished stimulating them.

Another way to sense the chakras in your body space is to rub your hands together and then place the palm of your positive hand (right hand if you're right-handed, left hand if you're left-handed) about three inches (8 cm) in front of each chakra gate.

Rubbing your hands together polarizes them slightly, making it easier for you to sense the resonance of each chakra consciously. If you begin by rubbing your hands together and then you place your positive hand above your first chakra gate, your palm will register its unique resonance.

To continue the process, remove your hand. Rub your hands together again and then place the palm of your positive hand in front of the second chakra gate. Your palm will register a slightly higher resonance than your first chakra. Continue in the same way by rubbing your palms together and experiencing the unique resonance of the third, fourth, fifth, sixth, and seventh chakras.

Once you've experienced the resonance of the seven traditional chakras, use the same technique to sense the resonance of your etheric, physical, and physical-material chakras.

After you've finished stimulating all thirteen chakras, take a few minutes to enjoy the effects you experience emotionally, mentally, and spiritually.

---

## Exercise: Activating a Chakra

Now that you can sense the chakras in your body space, you can take the next step in chakra healing by activating one of your chakras. You will learn the technique by activating your heart chakra. Afterward, you can use the same technique to activate any other chakra in your subtle energy system.

To activate your heart chakra, find a comfortable position with your back straight. Close your eyes and breathe yogically for two to three minutes. Then count backward from five to one and from ten to one. Use the standard method to relax your muscles and to center yourself in your subtle field of energy and consciousness.

When you're ready to continue, assert, "*It's my intent to activate my heart chakra.*" Once you've activated your heart chakra, you'll feel a glowing sensation along with a heightened sense of well-being. You can enhance these effects by asserting, "*It's my intent to turn my organs of perception inward on the level of my heart chakra.*" By turning your organs of perception inward, you'll become even more conscious of the shift that has taken place once your heart chakra is active. Remain centered in your subtle field with your attention focused on your heart chakra for fifteen minutes.

After fifteen minutes, you can return to normal consciousness by counting from one to five. When you reach the number five, open your eyes. You will feel wide awake, perfectly relaxed, and better than you did before. Repeat as needed.

---

### Exercise: Centering Yourself in a Chakra Field

After you've activated your heart chakra, the next step in chakra healing will be to center yourself in the corresponding chakra field. By centering yourself in the chakra field, your awareness will emerge directly from the reservoir of prana that animates you and the heart of every radiant person.

To center yourself in your heart chakra field, find a comfortable position with your back straight. Close your eyes and breathe yogically for two to three minutes. Count backward from five to one and from ten to one. Then use the standard method to relax your muscles and to center yourself in your subtle field of energy and consciousness. When you're ready to continue, assert, "*It's my intent to activate my heart chakra.*" Take a few moments to enjoy the effects. Then assert, "*It's my intent to center myself in my heart chakra field.*" You can enhance the effects by turning your organs of perception inward. To do that, assert, "*It's my intent to turn my organs of perception inward on the level of my heart chakra field.*" Remain centered in your heart chakra field for fifteen minutes.

After fifteen minutes, you can return to normal consciousness by counting from one to five. When you reach the number five, open your eyes. You will feel wide awake, perfectly relaxed, and better than you did before. Repeat as needed.

The same technique can be used to center yourself in any chakra field from the first to the one hundred and forty-sixth. Before you center yourself in a chakra field, however, it's important to activate the corresponding chakra gate.

---

## Exercise: Chakra Balancing

Another technique that will enhance the functions of your chakras and bring them into balance is called *chakra balancing*. By practicing the exercise regularly, not only will you increase the amount of healing energy you have available but you will also bring the energy into balance so that energy will be distributed evenly throughout your subtle field.

The best time to practice chakra balancing is the morning. I don't recommend practicing it around bedtime since it tends to stimulate the nerves and can keep you awake. If you practice the exercise regularly, you will soon begin to experience the effects; your energy level will increase, filling you with a greater sense of well-being, and you will enhance the amount of healing power you have available.

To begin chakra balancing, find a comfortable sitting position with your back straight. Then close your eyes and breathe yogically for two to three minutes. Count backward from five to one and from ten to one.

When you've reached the number one, repeat this affirmation to yourself in words, not thoughts: *"I'm deeply relaxed, feeling better than I did before."* Then assert, *"It's my intent to bring my mental attention to my first chakra at the base of my spine."* Almost immediately the chakra gate will begin to vibrate. The vibration emerges from the front of the chakra gate, making it easy to locate the chakra. Once the chakra has begun to vibrate, breathe into it so that the prana entering your subtle field on each inhalation activates the chakra further. Next, place the palm of your positive hand above the front of the chakra gate. For the first chakra, this will be a point between your legs about six inches (15 cm) below the perineum. For the second through sixth chakra, your hand will be two to three inches (5 to 8 cm) above the surface of your physical body. For the crown chakra, your hand will be two to three inches (5 to 8 cm) above the top of your head with the palm down above the chakra gate, which faces up.

Once you've activated the first chakra using your mental attention, your breath, and the palm of your positive hand, you will chant the universal *ohm* from the chakra three times, starting at the base of the spine and ending at the crown. Raise the *ohm* one note for each chakra, beginning with G for the first chakra, going through the seven notes of the scale (as you go through the seven chakras).

It's important to note that the tone you chant must cause a sympathetic vibration in the chakra. A sympathetic vibration in your chakra can be likened to the sympathetic vibration created in a violin string after a tuning fork in the same frequency has been struck next to it. After chanting from the seventh chakra, close your eyes and breathe normally through the nose for ten more minutes while you enjoy the positive effects the exercise has had on your subtle energy system and physical body.

## Summary

In this chapter, you learned how the chakras function and how they contribute to the health of your subtle field and physical body. Then you learned how to sense your chakras, activate a chakra gate, and center yourself in a chakra field. In chakra balancing, you learned to enhance and balance the flow of prana through the seven traditional chakras in your body space.

By activating and balancing the flow of prana through your chakras and by centering yourself in your chakra fields on a regular basis, you will bring your subtle energy system into a state of radiant good health. This will benefit you as a healer and enhance your ability to share pleasure, love, intimacy, and joy with other people.

In the next chapter, you will take chakra healing to the next level by using the chakras to heal yourself and another person. You will learn to fill a chakra field with prana and to perform chakra cleansing. After that you will learn to perform advanced chakra healing with color, using some of the knowledge you gained in chapters 5 and 6 on auric healing.

# Chapter 8
# Advanced Chakra Healing

In the last chapter you learned to activate your chakras and center your-self in your chakra fields. Then you learned to perform chakra balanc-ing. With the skills you now have, you're ready to fill your chakra fields with prana. By filling your chakra fields with prana, you will enhance their health and you will prepare them to participate in advanced chakra healing. Advanced chakra healing will enable you to heal ailments in body, soul, and spirit at their root in the subtle field.

---

### Exercise: Filling a Chakra Field with Prana

Filling a chakra field with prana is the foundation of advanced chakra healing. Once you've mastered the technique, you can use it to fill any chakra field with prana.

To begin the exercise, find a comfortable position with your back straight. Close your eyes and breathe yogically for two to three minutes. Then count backward from five to one and from ten to one. Use the standard method to relax your muscles and to center yourself in your subtle field of energy and conscious-ness. Then assert, *"It's my intent to activate my heart chakra."* Take a few moments to enjoy the effects. Then assert, *"It's my intent to center myself in my heart chakra field."*

You can enhance the effects by turning your organs of perception inward. To do that, assert, "*It's my intent to turn my organs of perception inward on the level of my heart chakra field.*" Enjoy the shift for a few moments. Then assert, "*It's my intent to fill my heart chakra field with prana.*" Don't do anything after that. Don't try to control your thoughts or enhance the flow of prana. Just let the healing energy fill your heart chakra field for the next fifteen minutes.

After fifteen minutes, you can return to normal consciousness by counting from one to five. When you reach the number five, open your eyes. You will feel wide awake, perfectly relaxed, and better than you did before.

Now that you've filled your heart chakra field with prana, you can enhance your skill by filling more than one chakra field with prana. There are several combinations that will provide you with tangible benefits. To increase your security, you can fill your first chakra field and third chakra field with prana. To enhance your joy, you can fill your second chakra field and fifth chakra field with prana, and to enhance your ability to perform chakra healing, you can fill your fourth chakra field and sixth chakra field with prana.

Once you've enhanced your ability to work with your own chakras, you can perform chakra cleansing first on yourself and then on another person.

## Chakra Cleansing

In *chakra cleansing*, you will use the prana that radiates through your chakra fields to cleanse the subtle energy system. You will perform the exercise on yourself first. Then you will perform the same exercise on another person.

Some healers use chakra cleansing as an integral part of each healing session. It can be used along with auric, pranic, and chakra healing and the techniques of laying on of hands. Always perform chakra cleansing on the front of the body and work down from the seventh chakra to the first chakra.

## Exercise: Chakra Cleansing

To perform chakra cleansing on yourself, find a comfortable position with your back straight. Then close your eyes and breathe yogically for two to three minutes. Count backward from five to one, then from ten to one. Then use the standard method to relax your muscles and to center yourself in your subtle field of energy and consciousness. Once you're centered, open your eyes but keep them slightly unfocused. Then use your masculine hand to make clockwise circular motions about six inches (15 cm) above the feminine pole of each chakra gate, beginning with your seventh chakra at the top of your head. Your palm should be facing the chakra and your fingers should be slightly extended. Make clockwise rotations (at a moderate pace) until you feel the chakra begin to vibrate.

Once your crown chakra has begun to vibrate, move your hand to your sixth chakra, at your brow, and repeat the process. Continue in the same way, making clockwise rotations above each chakra, until you reach your first chakra at the base of your spine. After you've stimulated all seven traditional chakras, close your eyes and take ten minutes to enjoy the effects. Then count from one to five. When you reach the number five, open your eyes. You will feel wide awake and perfectly relaxed, and you will experience the residual glow that comes from having cleansed your chakras.

## Exercise: Chakra Cleansing with a Partner

Once you've performed chakra cleansing on yourself, you can use a simple variation to perform chakra cleansing on another person. Always explain what you will be doing and answer your subject's questions before you begin. Then have your subject lie on their back with their arms at their sides. To help them relax, have them close their eyes and breathe deeply through the nose.

Once your subject is relaxed, close your eyes and begin to breathe yogically for two to three minutes. Then count backward, silently, from five to one and from ten to one. Use the standard method to relax your muscles and to center yourself in your subtle field of energy and consciousness. Then silently assert, "*It's my intent to center myself in my subtle field.*" Once you're centered, open your eyes but keep them slightly unfocused. Then rub your hands together for ten seconds to polarize them. After your hands are polarized, you will make the first of seven strokes with your positive hand over the front of your subject's seven traditional chakras.

The technique will work best if you keep the palm of your positive hand six inches (15 cm) above the surface of your subject's body. Do not work directly on the body since it will interfere with the polarity and natural sensitivity of your hands. At the beginning of each stroke, inhale through your nose and hold your breath. Then, with your fingers trailing behind your palm, make your first stroke down your subject's body. At the end of the stroke, exhale through your mouth. Then inhale through your nose and hold your breath while you make the next stroke. Repeat six more times until you've made seven strokes.

After you've completed seven strokes, use your masculine hand to make clockwise circular rotations above your subject's crown chakra, at the top of their head. Continue for two minutes at a moderate speed with your hand six inches (15 cm) above the chakra. After two minutes, move your hand to your subject's sixth chakra and repeat. Continue in the same way with your subject's fifth, fourth, third, second, and first chakras.

After working individually on the seven traditional chakras, rub your hands together again and make seven more strokes down the front of your subject's body with your positive hand.

When you're finished, close your eyes and recharge yourself. Then count from one to five and bring yourself out of the exercise. Give your subject an additional five minutes to enjoy the benefits of chakra cleansing. The additional time will allow him or her to sense the changes taking place and to integrate them into their subtle field.

Then count from one to five and have your subject open his or her eyes. After your subject is gone, rinse your hands in cold water to clear away any residual negative energy.

Chakra cleansing, like chakra balancing and yogic breathing, can be used to enhance good health and wellness. You can practice chakra cleansing any time on anyone you like, including your spouse, friends, and clients.

## Healing Rays and Emotions

Now that you've learned to fill your chakra fields with prana and to perform chakra cleansing, you have all the skills and experience necessary to perform chakra healing. Chakra healing can be used as a self-healing technique or to heal another person.

In the next exercise, you will perform an absentee healing on another person by projecting clear rays of healing energy to them from your fourth and sixth chakras (heart chakra and third eye). Then you will fill their etheric aura with prana. You can use the same technique for self-healing by visualizing an image of yourself on your visual screen.

---

### Exercise: Advanced Chakra Healing

In preparation for the session, get your client's permission and explain what you will be doing. Agree on a time for the healing and what ailment you'll be treating. It's important for your client to be relaxed during the session, so he or she should be in a place where there won't be disturbances by other people or electronic devices.

To begin advanced chakra healing, find a comfortable position with your back straight. Close your eyes and breathe yogically for two to three minutes. Then count backward from five to one and from ten to one. Use the standard method to relax your muscles and center yourself in your subtle field of energy and consciousness. Then assert, "*It's my intent to create a visual screen eight feet (2.5 m) in front of me.*" Continue by asserting, "*It's my intent to visualize* (subject's name here) *on my visual screen.*" Once he or she is on your screen, assert, "*It's my intent to activate my fourth chakra.*" Take a few moments to enjoy the shift. Then assert, "*It's my intent to center myself in my fourth chakra field.*"

When you're ready to continue, assert, "*It's my intent to activate my sixth chakra.*" Then assert, "*It's my intent to center myself in my sixth chakra field.*" Take two to three minutes to enjoy the shift. Then assert, "*It's my intent to fill my fourth chakra field with prana.*" Continue by asserting, "*It's my intent to fill my sixth chakra field with prana.*"

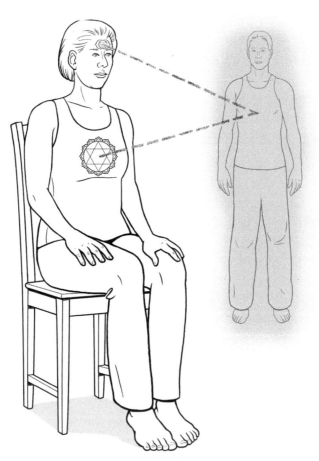

*Projecting Healing Rays*

By filling the chakra fields with prana, you will experience a glowing sensation emerging from the chakra gates. After a short time, the glowing sensation will grow more intense and you will experience pressure at the front of the chakra gates. Once you feel the pressure, assert, "*It's my intent to project rays of healing energy from my fourth and sixth chakras to the part of my client's body I've chosen to heal.*" The fourth and sixth chakras are used in advanced chakra healing because the heart chakra is an outward manifestation of the divine heart (Atman). And the rays projected from it will have a powerful healing effect. The sixth chakra is used because it's associated with the intuitive mind and the ability to view the subtle worlds of energy and consciousness.

Continue sending both rays for ten minutes. At the same time, feel your client absorb the rays into the diseased tissue. After ten minutes, visualize that the diseased tissue is perfectly healthy and glowing with energy. Then transfer the healing rays to your client's etheric aura. As the aura fills with prana, it will expand and begin to glow. Take two to three minutes to work on his or her aura. Then release the rays from your heart chakra and third eye. Release your client and your visual screen. Complete the session by recharging yourself.

Once your subtle field has been recharged, mentally affirm, "*Every time I perform a healing, I'm healed and I become a more effective channel for healing.*" Return to normal consciousness by counting from one to five. When you reach the number five, open your eyes. You will feel wide awake, perfectly relaxed, and better than you did before.

## Color Healing

There is a variation to advanced chakra healing called color healing. It's identical to advanced chakra healing except that the colored rays you project give the diseased tissue the exact dosage or vibration of energy it needs to be healed.

There are four major healing colors that can be use in color healing: yellow, green, blue, and violet. These colors have the most pronounced healing effect, although in some cases orange, red, and pink can be effective. The colors you project to your client must always be clear and bright. Never project colors that are dull, muddy, or dirty.

There are no rules for determining which healing color will most benefit a client. You must trust your intuition and treat each client individually. Your intuition will tell you which color is the appropriate one in a given situation.

Sometimes the appropriate color will appear spontaneously. If it does, continue to project it to your client. If no color spontaneously appears, then you will assert, *"It's my intent to project the rays in the appropriate healing color to heal my client."*

---

### Exercise: Chakra Healing with Color

In preparation for color healing, get your client's permission and observe the normal protocols for absentee healing. Then find a comfortable position with your back straight. Close your eyes and breathe yogically for two to three minutes. Count backward from five to one and from ten to one. Use the standard method to relax your muscles and center yourself in your subtle field of energy and consciousness.

When you're ready to continue, assert, *"It's my intent to create a visual screen about eight feet (2.5 m) in front of me."* Then assert, *"It's my intent to visualize* (subject's name here) *on my visual screen."* Once your client is on your screen, assert, *"It's my intent to activate my heart chakra."* Take a few moments to enjoy the shift. Then assert, *"It's my intent to center myself in my heart chakra field."* When you're ready to continue, assert, *"It's my intent to activate my sixth chakra."* Then assert, *"It's my intent to center myself in my sixth chakra field."*

Take two to three minutes to enjoy the changes you feel. Then assert, *"It's my intent to fill my heart chakra field with prana."* Continue by asserting, *"It's my intent to fill my sixth chakra field with prana.*" Once you feel pressure at the front of the chakra gates, assert, "*It's my intent to project rays of healing energy from my fourth and sixth chakras to the part of my client's body I've chosen to heal.*"

Feel your client absorb the healing rays into the diseased tissue. If a healing color doesn't spontaneously appear, assert, "*It's my intent to project the rays in the appropriate healing color to heal my client.*" If the healing color still doesn't appear, then your client doesn't require a specific color during the session. In that case, continue projecting clear rays into the diseased tissue.

Continue the healing for ten more minutes. Then visualize that the diseased tissue is perfectly healthy and glowing with energy. Continue by transferring the healing rays to your client's etheric aura. As the aura fills with prana, it will expand and begin to glow. Take two to three minutes to work on his or her aura. Then release the ray from your heart chakra and third eye. Release your client and your visual screen. Complete the session by recharging yourself.

When you are completely re-energized, mentally affirm, "*Every time I perform healing, I'm healed and I become a more effective channel for healing.*" Then return to normal consciousness by counting from one to five. When you reach the number five, open your eyes. You will feel wide awake, perfectly relaxed, and better than you did before.

## Summary

In this chapter, you learned to fill your chakra fields with prana and to perform chakra cleansing. Then you learned to perform advanced chakra healing and chakra healing with color.

In the next chapter, you will learn to perform mental healing. You will learn to use the prana brush and the prana box—two of the most powerful tools available to the spiritual healer. Afterward, you will combine the techniques of mental healing with the techniques you've learned earlier to heal some of the most common ailments that affect people in the modern world.

# Chapter 9
# Mental Healing

Mental healing includes remote viewing and healing visualizations within your client's body. As part of your healing visualizations, you will create tools that you can use to heal diseased organs and distorted fields of energy and consciousness.

Two tools that are particularly effective are the prana brush, which can be used to clean out diseased organs, and the prana box, which can be used along with the healing power of bliss to heal particularly stubborn ailments in both the subtle field and the physical body.

## Two Successful Case Histories

I've included two successful case histories in this chapter to give you an idea of how visualizations can be used in mental healing.

In the first case, I worked on a client who broke a leg while skiing. I was unable to see him in person, so all the work was done at a distance, on my visual screen. After using remote viewing to diagnose the problem, I mentally projected myself inside his body beside the fracture. I used my intent and mental attention to create tools to perform mental healing. They included a tube of glue, which I applied to both ends of the broken bone. When the glue began to harden, I squeezed the two ends together and held them until the glue set and the bone was firmly reconnected. Then I mixed a plaster compound and applied it to the seam where I had connected the two bones. After it hardened, I created a file that I used to sand the area so that it was perfectly smooth. Finally,

I created a tube labeled "healing medicine." I applied the medicine to the crack and then rubbed the medicine in, all the time radiating healing energy through my hands into the bone. I completed the healing by visualizing that the bone was completely healed. The reports I received later confirmed that the bone healed in record time.

In the other case, I worked on a baby who'd fallen down a flight of stairs. When I was asked to work on her, she was in critical condition. The child had torn ligaments in the back of her neck. She was bleeding internally and had multiple blood clots in the arteries and veins of her neck and head.

I began the session by visualizing myself inside one of the clogged vessels. I created an electric drill, which I used to break up the blood clots in her neck. When the clots were broken into small pieces, I visualized myself sweeping them up and putting them in a bucket. I went from one blood vessel to the next until all were unclogged. Then I began working on the torn ligaments and muscles. I repaired them by sewing the ripped ends together. I imagined that I had a needle and thread with me and sewed together each ligament and each torn muscle. Finally, I returned to the blood vessels and applied "healing medicine" to the ones I had repaired. I did the same with the muscles and ligaments, applying medicine to each one I'd sewn together. This procedure took me more than two hours, but it was well worth it because the next day I was informed the baby was out of danger and was making a rapid recovery.

Two new techniques that have proven to be particularly effective are the prana brush and the prana box. You will learn how they function now. Later in this chapter, you will use them along with the traditional techniques of mental healing to heal some of the most common diseases afflicting people today.

## The Prana Brush

The prana brush is an extremely effective tool because it radiates prana when you brush it against a diseased organ. Since the distorted energy that supports disease (energy with individual qualities) and healing energy in the form of prana (energy with universal qualities) cannot occupy the same space at the same time, brushing the diseased tissue or the organ with a prana brush releases the distorted energy and replaces it with life-affirming energy.

The prana brush can be used on the skin to heal skin disease or inside the body to heal any organ or tissue that requires your attention. Always brush the outside of the diseased organ or tissue first. Then visualize yourself inside the organ and/or tissue and brush it from the inside until prana has replaced the distorted energy that was the foundation of disease.

## The Prana Box

The prana box is one of the most powerful tools available to the healer. It combines the healing power of prana with the overwhelming healing power of consciousness in the form of bliss.

For millennia, healers have recognized that there are three forces in the universe. Energy with individual qualities has the power to cause disease, but it's the weakest of the three forces. Healing energy in the form of prana is stronger and can release energy with individual qualities when used effectively, no matter how dense and distorted it has become. The strongest force by far is consciousness in the form of bliss. Most healers use prana to perform healing. However, the most successful healers have always used consciousness—usually in combination with prana—to heal themselves and their clients.

---

### Exercise: Mental Healing on Yourself with a Prana Brush

Before you use mental healing and the prana brush to heal yourself, choose a physical ailment you wish to heal. Then find a comfortable position with your back straight. Close your eyes and breathe yogically for two to three minutes. Then use the standard method to relax your muscles and center yourself in your subtle field of energy and consciousness.

Continue by asserting, "*It's my intent to create a visual screen eight feet (2.5 m) in front of me.*" Then assert, "*It's my intent to visualize an image of myself on my visual screen."* Take two to three minutes to scan the front and back of your body. If you're attracted to any particular part of your body, it's an indication that distorted energy is present. Take note of that and the rightness or wrongness of the vibration. Then project yourself next to the image of yourself on the screen. Use your hand to scan your body for another two to three minutes.

When you're satisfied with what you've learned, assert, *"It's my intent to project myself inside my body, standing next to the body part I've chosen to heal."* Use all your appropriate senses to examine the body part. Feel the wobbles in its vibration; check the texture, temperature, and finally color. Diseased tissue is usually dark in color and has an irregular texture and shape. Often the tissue will look lumpy or feel too cold or too hot.

When you're satisfied with what you've learned, create your healing tools. You can create doctor's tools, kitchen tools, mechanic's tools, or painter's tools. In mental healing, any tools will do, even tools like ray guns that exist only on the mental plane. Then begin healing the diseased tissue from the outside. You can create more tools if you need them. If it's appropriate, you can mentally project yourself inside the diseased tissue and continue the healing there.

When you've completed working with your tools, release them and visualize that you're holding a prana brush. Use it to release any distorted energy that remains and to saturate the body part with prana. When you're finished, release the prana brush. Then visualize that the body part is perfectly healthy and radiating prana freely. Mentally project yourself back to your original position next. Then release the image of yourself and the visual screen. Count from one to five. Then open your eyes and bring yourself out of the healing exercise.

## Exercise: Mental Healing on Another Person with a Prana Box

In this exercise, you will use remote viewing to diagnose your client's condition. Then you will use the traditional techniques of mental healing and the prana box to heal them. In preparation for mental healing, get your client's permission and observe the normal protocols for absentee healing.

When you're ready to begin, find a comfortable position with your back straight. Then close your eyes and breathe yogically for two to three minutes. Use the standard method to relax your muscles and center yourself in your subtle field of energy and consciousness.

When you're ready to continue, assert, "*It's my intent to create a visual screen eight feet (2.5 m) in front of me.*" Then assert, "*It's my intent to visualize* (client's name here) *on the screen in front of me.*"

Scan your client's body, paying particular attention to the rightness or wrongness of his or her vibration. When you're ready to continue, assert, "*It's my intent to project myself on the screen next to my client.*" Continue your scan for two to three minutes. Then assert, "*It's my intent to project myself inside my client's body by the area I've agreed to heal.*" Examine the body part from the outside and then from the inside. When you're satisfied with what you've learned, create a set of healing tools. Then begin healing the diseased tissue. You can create more tools if you need them. If it's appropriate, mentally project yourself inside the diseased tissue and continue the healing there. Take your time and be thorough. When you're satisfied with your work, release your tools and get ready to perform the orgasmic bliss mudra.

To do this mudra, place the tip of your tongue on your upper palette and bring it straight back until it comes to rest at the point where the hard palette rolls up and becomes soft. Once the tip of your tongue is in that position, put the bottom of your feet together so that the soles are touching. Then bring your hands in front of your solar plexus and place the inside tips of your thumbs together. Continue by bringing the outsides of your index fingers together from the tips to the first joint. Next, bring the outsides of your middle fingers together from the first to the second joint. The fourth and fifth fingers should be curled into your palm.

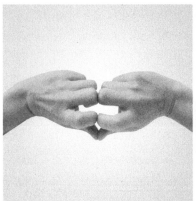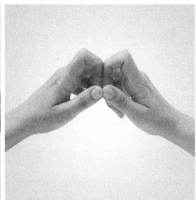

*The Orgasmic Bliss Mudra*

Once your tongue, fingers, and feet are in position, hold the mudra while you mentally create a prana box that surrounds the diseased organ or tissue you wish to heal. The size and shape of the box should closely follow the contours of the diseased tissue.

To construct the box, assert, *"It's my intent to create a prana box around the diseased organ (or tissue) I've chosen to heal."* Once you can sense and/or see the box, assert, *"It's my intent to fill the box with bliss and release all the distorted matter, energy, and consciousness within it."* Don't do anything after that. Bliss will fill the box you've created and release the distorted fields permanently.

Some of you may experience a sense of relief and/or a pop when bliss fills the box. Both indicate that the distorted fields within the box have been released and bliss has filled the empty space.

Once the distorted fields have been released, release the prana box and the orgasmic bliss mudra. Then take a few moments to recharge yourself. When you feel your subtle field glowing with energy, count from one to five. When you reach the number five, open your eyes. You will feel wide awake, perfectly relaxed, and better than you did before.

## Healing Solutions for Common Ailments

In the following section, you will use the techniques you already learned and additional mudras and techniques to heal common ailments. Once you're confident in your ability, you can adapt these techniques to heal additional ailments. Let your intuition be your guide and use the techniques you've mastered in this chapter and earlier chapters to enhance you health and well-being and the health and well-being of your clients.

### Abdominal Cramps for Women

Abdominal cramps can be so painful that they can disable a woman. In order to overcome them, a healer can use remote viewing to locate the distorted fields of matter, energy, and consciousness responsible for them. These fields will be particularly dense and active. To release them, perform the *Mental Healing on Another Person with a Prana Box* exercise on page 111. If you are healing yourself, follow the *Mental Healing on Yourself with a Prana Brush* exercise on page 109. On the same day, practice the *abdominal relief mudra* and continue to perform it for six more days. On the seventh day, use remote viewing to find out if any of the original distorted energy remains. If it does, repeat the entire process one more time.

---

### Exercise: The Abdominal Relief Mudra

This mudra will enhance the flow of prana through the chakras that supply the abdomen with prana. These chakras include the second chakra, the lower etheric chakra, the lower physical chakra, and the lower physical-material chakra. The mudra also stimulates the acupuncture point in the colon, which releases prana from the first chakra and stimulates the Kundalini Shakti—one of the most powerful forms of energy in the subtle energy field.

To begin the abdominal relief mudra, find a comfortable position with your back straight. Then close your eyes and breathe deeply through the nose for two to three minutes. Continue by placing the tips of your index fingers together. Then place the tips of your thumbs together. Bend the middle fingers, ring fingers, and pinky of each hand into the palms and apply a little pressure to the mound of Venus (the base of your thumb) with your curled fingertips. Hold the mudra for ten minutes and repeat every day for seven days.

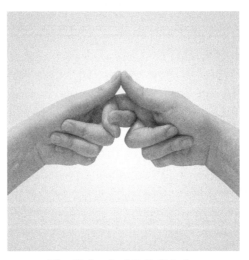

*The Abdominal Relief Mudra*

*Burnout*

In a healthy person, the authentic mind plays the dominant role and the individual mind and ego support it. In extreme situations, like burnout, it's possible for the individual mind and ego to usurp the functions of the authentic mind and to function as a surrogate mind. When this happens, you will find yourself alienated from yourself on the mental level. The mind will become chaotic without the ability to focus, concentrate, or form an authentic and stable identity. Without a stable identity, it will become increasingly difficult for a person to feel or express their authentic feelings and emotions.

---

### Exercise: Healing Burnout

Healing burnout is a four-step process.

**Step 1:** Let go of restrictive beliefs. Most people hold on to a number of beliefs that restrict their activities and prevent prana from flowing freely. Examples of restrictive beliefs are:

*"I have to be perfect all the time and in all situations."*

*"I have to be in control of every aspect of my life."*

*"It is not enough to be myself and to radiate prana through my body, soul, and spirit."*

To let go of a restrictive belief, relax and center yourself by using the yogic breath and the standard method. Then visualize an image of yourself on your visual screen. Continue by asserting, *"It's my intent to see the distorted fields in my subtle field that support the restrictive belief I want to release."* As soon as you see the fields of distorted matter, energy, and consciousness, assert, *"It's my intent to surround each distorted field I'm viewing with a prana box."* Then perform the orgasmic bliss mudra. Continue to hold it while you fill the prana box with bliss and release the distorted fields.

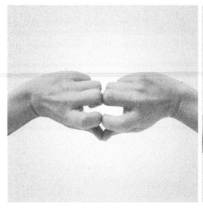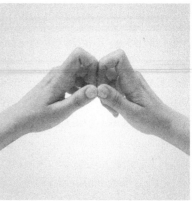

*The Orgasmic Bliss Mudra*

Repeat the same exercise every day until all the distorted fields that supported the restrictive belief are gone. You can repeat the process with as many restrictive beliefs as you want or until you feel your authentic identity begin to reemerge.

**Step 2:** Strengthen your boundaries. Boundaries include chakra fields, the surfaces of your resource fields, and the surfaces of the auric fields that surround your subtle field. To keep your surface boundaries strong, detach yourself from people who don't respect your personal space and who inhibit you from being yourself and/or expressing yourself freely and honestly.

**Step 3:** Give up unhealthy attachments. Most unhealthy attachments that contribute to burnout are created by energetic intrusions. Intrusions create dependency and block your access to prana. In chapter 12, you will find exercises designed specifically to release intrusions so that you can once again be yourself and express yourself without being blocked or manipulated by distorted fields of matter, energy, and consciousness.

**Step 4:** Enhance the flow of prana through your energy field. To enhance the flow of prana through your subtle field, perform the prana mudra. Practice the mudra every day for two weeks. If symptoms persist, repeat the four-step process again.

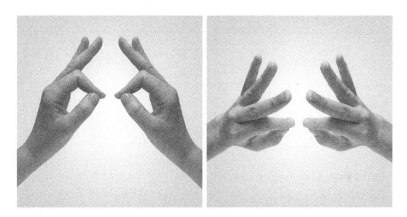

*The Prana Mudra*

## Cancer

To heal cancer, it's essential to do four things: heal the tumors, release the distorted fields that support them, strengthen the immunological system, and enhance the flow of prana through the subtle field and physical body.

To heal the tumor, you will use the techniques of mental healing with the prana brush on page 109. To release the distorted fields that support the tumor, you will use the prana box (go to page 111). To strengthen the immunological system, you will perform the *empowerment mudra*.

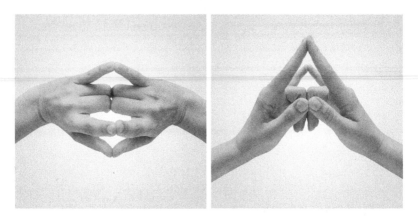

*The Empowerment Mudra*

And to enhance the flow of prana through the subtle field, you will perform the prana mudra.

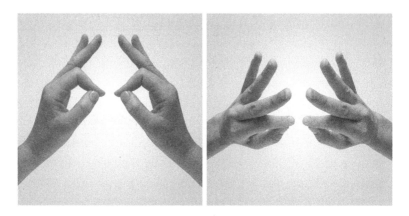

*The Prana Mudra*

**Days 1–7:** In the mornings of the first seven days, you will heal the tumors and release the distorted fields that supported them. To do that, use the yogic breath and the standard method to relax and center yourself in your subtle field. Then visualize your client on your visual screen. Continue by projecting yourself inside their body. Visualize the tools you will use to heal the tumor. Heal one tumor at a time. Complete each process by using the prana brush to saturate the area where the tumor(s) was located with prana. Next, project yourself back to your original position and surround the distorted fields that supported each tumor with a prana box. Perform the orgasmic bliss mudra. Then fill the prana box with bliss and release the distorted fields. Complete the healing by recharging yourself. Then bring yourself out of the session by counting from one to five.

In the evenings on the first seven days, you will use the yogic breath and the standard method to relax and center yourself in your subtle field. Then you will visualize your client on your visual screen. You will fill your own etheric aura with prana. Then you will use auric healing and gazing to fill your client's etheric aura with prana.

**Days 8–19:** In the mornings of days eight through nineteen, you will have your client perform the *empowerment mudra*. In the evenings, you will have your client perform the prana mudra.

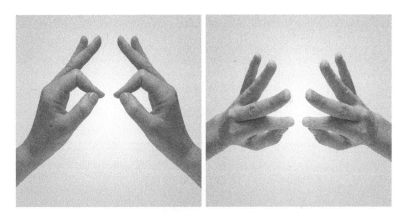

*The Prana Mudra*

---

### Exercise: The Empowerment Mudra

To perform this mudra, find a comfortable position with your back straight. Breathe deeply through the nose for two to three minutes. Then place the tip of your tongue directly behind the point where your teeth meet your upper gums. Put the outside tips of your thumbs together to form a triangle. Then put the tips of your index fingers together to form the second triangle. Once the tips of your index fingers are touching, put the outsides of your middle and ring fingers together from the first to the second joint. Then put the inside tips of your pinkies together to form a third triangle.

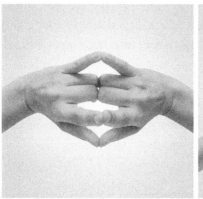 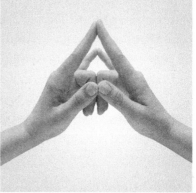

*The Empowerment Mudra*

When you look down at your hands, you will see three triangles. The first triangle has been created by your thumbs. The second triangle has been created by your index fingers, and the third triangle has been created by your pinkies. Hold the mudra for ten minutes with your eyes closed. Then release it and open your eyes.

Since cancer is so closely related to a person's worldview and sense of self, you can repeat this process until you feel that the cancer is gone and the underlying causes have been overcome.

## Depression

Depression is a form of repressed anger that can afflict anyone—even children. To heal depression, you will use remote viewing to locate the distorted fields that are the foundation of the problem. Then you will use mental healing and the prana box to release them. Afterward, you will use chakra cleansing to enhance the functions of the client's subtle field. You will also use the prana mudra, which can be used by your client to heal any residual effects.

---

### Exercise: Healing Depression

To begin, examine the auric field. Give special attention to the area surrounding the second chakra, because depression is related to suppressed anger and the second chakra regulates the ability to express anger freely without blame getting in the way. If you find distorted fields anywhere near the second chakra, or you feel a vibration that radiates depressed feelings or ideas, then perform the healing regimen that follows.

Every morning for seven days, perform chakra cleansing (see chapter 8). In the evening, fill the etheric aura with prana (see chapter 5). On the eighth day, surround any distorted fields of matter, energy, or consciousness that remains with a prana box and use bliss to release them (go to page 111). Then perform the prana mudra for ten minutes every day for ten days until you're satisfied that the depression has been relieved.

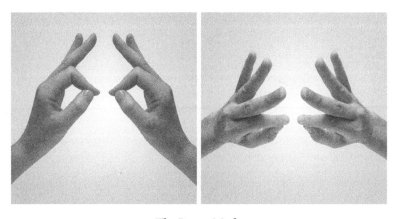

*The Prana Mudra*

## Hyperactivity

Hyperactivity is caused by a lack of balance within the subtle field. When there is too much pressure in one part of the subtle field, balance will be disrupted and the symptoms associated with hyperactivity will appear. In most cases, the pressure will be most severe at either the front or back of one or more chakra gates. To heal hyperactivity, it's best to treat it as both an acute and chronic problem. The first step will be to overcome the acute symptoms. The second step will be to create a regimen of energy work to heal the chronic problem and overcome the underlying issues.

---

### Exercise: Healing Hyperactivity

**Step 1:** To overcome the acute problems, you will use the yogic breath and the standard method to relax and center yourself in your subtle field. Then use the visual screen and remote viewing to study the condition of the thirteen chakra gates in body space. Take note of where you find fields of distorted energy that are in direct contact with the chakra gates. It's these fields that must be released first. To do that, you will use the prana box (go to page 111).

Once you've released the distorted fields that have disrupted a particular chakra gate, you will use chakra healing to fill the corresponding chakra field with prana (see chapter 8). Repeat the process for three days. Then use the same process to bring other chakras that have been blocked by distorted fields into balance. Recharge yourself at the end of each session. Then count from one to five and bring yourself out of the healing exercise.

**Step 2:** In step two, you, or your client, will perform the prana mudra every day, for two weeks. During the same time, you, or your client, can perform chakra cleansing on the subtle field every second day (see chapter 8).

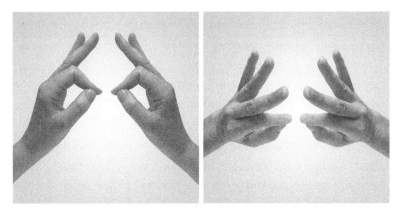

*The Prana Mudra*

## Kidney Stones

Kidney stones can create both an acute and chronic medical condition that can debilitate a person. In many cases, the pain associated with kidney stones is unbearable. In order to heal kidney stones, you will use a combination of mental healing, the prana brush, the prana box, and chakra healing.

---

### Exercise: Healing Kidney Stones

**Day 1:** To begin, use the yogic breath and standard method to relax and to center yourself in your subtle field. Then visualize an image of yourself (or your client) on your visual screen. Use remote viewing to diagnose the underlying problem. Then project yourself inside your body or your client's body. Create the appropriate tools to break up the stones and to painlessly remove them. Next, use the prana box to release the distorted fields that supported the ailment (go to page 111). Finally, use your prana brush to saturate your kidneys with prana (go to page 109). To complete the healing, visualize that the kidney is perfectly healthy and glowing with energy. Then release the screen and recharge yourself. After that, count from one to five and bring yourself out of the exercise.

**Days 2–7:** For the next six days, use the yogic breath and the standard method to relax and to center yourself in your subtle field. Then visualize an image of yourself (or your client) on your visual screen. Visualize yourself on the screen. Then place your assertive hand on one side of a kidney and your receptive hand opposite it. Use chakra healing with the minor energy centers in your palms to fill both kidneys with healing energy. Complete the process by visualizing that the kidneys are perfectly healthy and glowing with energy. Then release your client and the screen and recharge yourself. After that, count from one to five and bring yourself out of the exercise.

### Ulcerative Colitis

Colitis is a psychosomatic condition that has its foundation in the subtle field. It occurs when one of more chakras have become overburdened by distorted fields of energy and consciousness. In the case of colitis, it is the first chakra as well as the lower physical and physical-material chakras that have become overburdened by distorted fields of energy and consciousness.

---

### Exercise: Healing Ulcerative Colitis

To overcome the acute problems, you will use the yogic breath and the standard method to relax and center yourself in your subtle field. Then you will use the visual screen and remote viewing to study the condition of the first chakra gate as well as the lower physical and physical-material chakra gates.

Take note of where you find fields of distorted energy and consciousness that interact directly with the chakra gates. Then fill the first chakra field, lower physical chakra field, and lower physical-material fields with prana (go to chapter 5). Once they're glowing with prana, use the prana box to release the distorted fields of energy and consciousness that interfere with the functions of the first chakra gate, physical chakra gate, and physical-material chakra gate (go to page 111).

Next, use your remote viewing skills to observe the condition of the lower pelvic area. Use rays of energy from your fourth and sixth chakra to fill the area with the appropriate healing color (see chapter 8). Then use the prana brush to saturate the area with prana (go to page 109). Repeat the sessions for five days. At the end of each day's session, recharge yourself.

## Summary

In this chapter, you learned to perform mental healing and to use the prana brush and prana box to perform absentee healing. Then you learned to use a combination of healing techniques to heal common ailments such as cancer, hyperactivity, depression, colitis, etc. You can use many of the same techniques to heal other conditions that affect your health and the health of your clients.

So-called psychosomatic diseases are some of the easiest conditions to heal. Psychosomatic diseases include migraines, neurodermitis, phobias, ulcers, as well as many other diseases that influence people in the modern world. Diseases that are more closely related to weaknesses or a breakdown in the physical body such as heart disease, diabetes, and glandular problems can also be treated, but they often take more time before noticeable improvements appear. In both cases, however, use what you learned with confidence. If you work methodically and persistently, in time both you and your clients will benefit greatly from your work.

In the next chapter, you will learn to use vibration, empathy, and stroking in combination with what you've already learned to perform laying on of hands.

## Chapter 10

# Laying On of Hands

Everywhere you turn, history gives evidence of spiritual healing through the "laying on of hands." It's often used in combination with other techniques, such as anointing with oils, magnetizing cloth, cotton, water, and other natural substances. Sometimes direct contact is made with saliva and clay as described in the New Testament:

> "As Jesus passed by, he saw a man who was blind from his birth ... he spat on the ground, and made clay of the spittle, and anointed the eyes of the blind man with clay and said unto him, 'Go, wash in the pool of Siloam' ... he went his way, therefore, and washed, and came seeing." [16]

Sometimes the healing is done directly when the healer touches the client's physical body. But the healer can also work on the client's etheric aura without making physical contact. Usually, it's the healer who does the touching, but this is not always the case. The client can initiate the healing by touching the healer, or simply by coming within the healer's auric field. This remarkable healing from the New Testament will illustrate:

> "And a certain woman, which had an issue of blood twelve years, and had suffered many things of many physicians, and had spent

---

16. John 9:1–7 (KJV).

*all that she had, and was nothing bettered, but rather grew worse, when she had heard of Jesus, came in the crowd behind, and touched his garment. For she said, 'If I may touch but his clothes, I shall be whole.' And straightway the fountain of her blood was dried up, and she felt in her body that she was healed of that plague. And Jesus... turned him about in the crowd, and said, 'Daughter, thy faith hath made thee whole; go in peace and be whole of the plague.'"* [17]

## History of Laying On of Hands

For centuries, laying on of hands has been the preferred method of most spiritual healers. Evidence of its practice has been traced back more than fifteen thousand years to Neolithic cave paintings in the Pyrenees. Healing by direct contact, or what we call laying on of hands, appears to be a universal human practice. In ancient Egypt, laying on of hands was practiced from the earliest times, being the domain of the temple priests. Scholars and Egyptologists have found representations of direct healing on sarcophagi, jewelry, and wall paintings. Even to this day, we can see laying on of hands as part of the healing practices of the Rosicrucians and Masons, both of whom trace their lineage back to ancient Egypt.

The early Greeks were aware that a sick person could be healed through the laying on of hands. Hippocrates tells us, "*It is believed by many experienced doctors that the heat which oozes out of the hand, on being applied to the sick, is highly salutary and assuaging.*" [18]

It's only in the West, with the beginning of the Industrial Revolution and the Age of Reason, that the laying on of hands fell into disrepute. Even so, small groups like the Theosophists and Pentecostals have kept the tradition alive. Healings have continued unabated in these and other sects, sometimes spilling over into the general population.

---

17. Mark 5:30–35 (KJV).
18. Hippocrates, *Breaths, Book One [Liber de flatibus]*.

In this chapter, you will learn to perform the laying on of hands by combining the techniques of empathetic healing, vibrational healing, and stroking.

## Conditions for Laying On of Hands

Laying on of hands should be practiced in a quiet, serene environment where there are no disruptions. You should put aside sufficient time to talk to your client and explain the techniques you will be using before each healing session. In addition, you should allow your client to unburden him- or herself before the healing. It's highly unlikely that anyone suffering physically would be free from emotional and mental distress. Remember there is always a direct connection between good health and the client's psychological state.

After you've explained the techniques you will be using and what your client should expect, explain that healing energy can be experienced in different ways. It can be experienced as intense heat coming from the healer's hands, but it can also be experienced as "cold rays." Some clients feel a tingle or vibration in the area the healer is touching. Sometimes the tingling sensations run through the extremities. The client sometimes feels very light-headed or dizzy or becomes momentarily disoriented. In some cases, the client will feel nothing unusual except a deep sense of relaxation. After you've explained everything, have your client lie down and close his or her eyes. Then have them breathe deeply through the nose and relax. After you've met these conditions, you can begin the healing session.

## Preparing Yourself for Laying On of Hands

Before you make direct contact with your client, make sure you're in the right state to be an effective healing channel. I ensure this by breathing yogically and integrating the energy in Hara with my strong center in my subtle energy system. Only then will I place my hands on the client.

I recommend that you begin laying on of hands by working (placing your hands) on your client's head. Perform a general healing for about five minutes using prana healing and auric healing through the minor energy centers in your hands (see chapter 6). Then move your hands to the diseased part of your client's body and work there for about fifteen minutes using a combination of healing techniques, which should include vibrational and empathetic healing (you will learn both techniques in this chapter).

Other techniques can be useful, including chakra healing and mental healing. After you've finished working on the diseased area, bring your hands back to your client's head and use auric healing with your hands to fill his or her etheric aura with prana. After that, you can perform chakra cleansing, and you can recharge yourself.

In the following pages, you will learn to perform a complete session of laying on of hands. We will begin our study with vibrational healing.

## The Importance of Vibration

Many healers are consciously aware of a healing vibration running through their subtle field. I call it the central pranic vibration. The strength of the central pranic vibration and its efficacy in healing is directly related to the amount of prana flowing through the healer's subtle energy system and the amount of empathy the healer has for themselves and their client.

I've observed that students performing vibrational healing have a clearer, brighter, and larger auric field—a clear sign that more prana is radiating through it. Students performing vibrational healing for the first time have reported that they feel light-headed and their chakras glowed brightly. Others have told me that they felt their aura get bigger and warmer or that they felt their head grew larger once they achieved the vibrational state.

A stronger vibrational state with its increased energy level makes it possible for the healer to channel vast amounts of healing energy directly through his or her hands. That's why it's not unusual for vibrational healing to have an immediate effect on the client.

## Exercise: Achieving the Vibrational State

You can quickly achieve the vibrational state by practicing the following breathing exercise. To begin, find a comfortable position with your back straight. Then begin to breathe deeply through your nose without separation between inhalation and exhalation. Continue by asserting, "*It's my intent to activate my heart chakra.*" Then assert, "*It's my intent to center myself in my heart chakra field.*" Take two to three minutes to enjoy the shift. Then pay attention to the rhythms of your body and how your feelings influence them. Once you can clearly sense your bodily rhythms, allow them to direct the rhythm of your breath. As soon as the rhythms become synchronized—and your breath, feelings, and physical sensations are in union—bring your mental attention to your hands. Continue to breathe without separation between inhalation and exhalation, but strengthen both inhalation and exhalation (so that they're a bit forced) until you feel your hands become warm and begin to vibrate. After that, relax and breathe normally again.

After a short time, which could be from thirty seconds to five minutes, depending on how adept you are at this technique, you will begin to feel a deep, almost overwhelming compassion for your client. This will trigger the central pranic vibration, which will begin in the central cavity of your body.

You will recognize the central pranic vibration because it will be more subtle than the original vibration in your hands. That vibration will wear off as soon as you relax your breathing. In contrast, the central pranic vibration will radiate outward from the central cavity of your body into your hands, and it will continue for as long as you pay attention to it. When it reaches your hands and replaces the original vibration, you're ready to perform vibrational healing. Enjoy the vibration for five minutes longer. Then count from one to five and bring yourself out of the exercise. Repeat as needed.

Although vibrational healing can be used alone to heal ailments in body, soul, and spirit, it's most effective when it's used along with empathetic healing during a session of laying on of hands.

## Empathetic Healing

Although empathetic healing is the most important and powerful method of healing, I left it for last because, unlike prana healing, auric healing, chakra healing, etc., in empathetic healing the healer transcends his or her sense of individuality and reunites with the ultimate source of healing, Universal Consciousness. The temporary loss of personal identity can be a challenge, but it allows the healer to experience disease the same way the client does (although in a temporary and far milder form). For a short time, the healer feels the client's feelings, experiences the client's bodily sensations, and shares the client's thoughts.

We can say with some justification that in empathetic healing, the healer intercedes on behalf of the client by letting Universal Consciousness merge with him, and through him with his client. Since Universal Consciousness is a singularity, once union is achieved, there will be no place for duality, and, therefore, no place for disease to interfere with the universal qualities of radiant good health. The case history that follows illustrates just how immediate and powerful empathetic healing can be.

In an unusual case, a spontaneous healing resulted from empathetic healing. It occurred in one of my seminars while I demonstrated empathetic healing on a young woman who volunteered to be my subject. After the seminar, I spoke with her and she told me that a week before the seminar she'd visited a fertility clinic. The doctors who examined her recommended that she have an additional checkup at another clinic. Doctors at the second clinic discovered a nodule on the upper left side of her lung. X-rays from three years earlier were compared to the current x-rays, so the presence of the nodule was definitely confirmed. The doctors had decided a CAT scan would be necessary to obtain more information as to where this nodule was located and the consistency of it.

In the interim, she volunteered to be my subject for empathetic healing. This was two weeks after the discovery of the lung nodule. The scan had been cancelled due to failure of equipment and was postponed a week. While she was under the scanner a week later, the doctor in charge confirmed that nothing had shown up and the lung was clear.

She confided in me that during the empathic healing she had actually felt the warmth of the healing energy radiating through her. And that the left side of her body (where the nodule was) even seemed to be floating in the air, while the right side was still on the couch.

She was convinced that a healing actually occurred by the dizziness she felt afterward. She thanked me for my work and told me that it saved her from a painful and expensive operation and helped confirm her belief in spiritual healing and the spiritual aspects of life.

## The Three Fields of Empathy

For the healer, empathy is both a function of character and an integral part of their subtle field. In fact, the energy that supports empathy emerges from a resource field known as the field of empathy. The condition of this resource field has a direct effect on a person's level of empathy and their ability to use empathy in healing.

The field of empathy, like all resource fields, provides your subtle field with energy and consciousness. What's special about the field of empathy is that when functioning healthfully it will also become a compassionate healing space where you and your clients can meet energetically. The field of empathy can create that space because it provides the healer with a medium through which energy can be exchanged selflessly without the "I" or the ego getting in the way. The field of empathy has three parts: the personal field of empathy, the public field of empathy, and the transcendent field of empathy.

In order to heal yourself, heal other people, or heal your relationship to the source of healing, you must center yourself in the appropriate field of empathy. To heal yourself, you will center yourself in the personal field of empathy. To heal another person, you will center yourself in the public field of empathy. And to use your healing space to heal your relationship to the source of healing—Universal Consciousness—you will center yourself in the transcendent field of empathy.

Although empathy is a normal human attribute, and every human being has empathy, it's important for the healer to enhance their empathy to perform empathetic healing on themselves, their clients, and their relationship to Universal Consciousness. In order to do that, I've developed an exercise that uses resonance and the power of the universal sound *ohm*. As you learned in chapter 7, *ohm* is the sound of the universal vibration. This was the sound uttered by the universe at the moment of creation. It's also the sound of the life force that continues to animate all living beings.

Practice the exercise that follows every day for two weeks and your empathy will increase. So will your ability to successfully perform empathetic healing.

---

### Exercise: Resonating to Enhance Empathy

To begin the exercise, find a comfortable position with your back straight. Close your eyes and breathe yogically for two to three minutes. Then count backward from five to one and from ten to one. Use the standard method to relax your muscles and to center yourself in your subtle field of energy and consciousness. Then assert, "*It's my intent to center myself in my three fields of empathy.*" Continue by asserting, "*It's my intent to turn my organs of perception inward on the level of my three fields of empathy.*" Take a few moments to enjoy the shift. Then assert, "*It's my intent to fill my three fields of empathy with prana and pure consciousness.*" When you're ready to resonate, inhale into your healing space (the three fields of empathy). When you exhale, chant *ohm*.

Synchronize the sound you make with the vibration that emanates from the field of empathy. If you do, you will feel that *ohm* emerges directly from the field of empathy. As you continue to chant, allow the prana and consciousness from your healing space to radiate through your physical body and subtle field. In a short time, you will feel that the *ohm* you're chanting has become the singular expression of what you're experiencing and feeling. It's not necessary to chant too loudly, but it is best when you chant audibly. Continue chanting for about ten minutes. After ten minutes, bring yourself out of the exercise by counting from one to five.

The effects of resonating, especially after you've been doing it for a few days, will be profound. Resonating will create an ever-growing field of empathy. By returning to it regularly and strengthening it through resonating, empathy will become a resource that will enhance your life and relationships and make you an even more effective healer. Repeat as needed.

---

## Exercise: Empathetic Self-Healing

Now that you've learned to increase your empathy through resonating, you're ready to perform empathetic healing on yourself. To do that, choose an ailment you wish to heal. Then find a comfortable position with your back straight. Close your eyes and breathe yogically for two to three minutes. Then count backward from five to one and from ten to one. Use the standard method to relax your muscles and to center yourself in your subtle field of energy and consciousness.

When you're ready to continue, assert, "*It's my intent to center myself in my personal field of empathy.*" Continue by asserting, "*It's my intent to turn my organs of perception inward on the level of my personal field of empathy.*" Next assert, "*It's my intent to fill my personal field of empathy with prana and pure consciousness.*" Take a few moments to enjoy the shift. Then assert, "*It's my intent that healing energy and consciousness radiate through my personal field of empathy into the area of my body I've chosen to heal.*" Don't do anything after that. Just enjoy the process.

Take fifteen minutes to perform the healing. After fifteen minutes, visualize that the body part you chose to heal is glowing with radiant good health. Then count from one to five, open your eyes and bring yourself out of the exercise. Repeat as needed.

---

### Exercise: Healing Another Person with Empathy

Before you perform empathic healing on your client, explain what you will be doing and answer his or her questions. Decide on an ailment to be healed. Then have your client sit facing you about ten feet (3 m) away. When you're satisfied that your client is comfortable, have them close their eyes and breathe deeply through the nose. Then close your eyes and breathe yogically for two to three minutes. Count backward from five to one and from ten to one. Then use the standard method to relax your muscles and to center yourself in your subtle field of energy and consciousness.

When you're ready to continue, assert, "*It's my intent to center myself in my public field of empathy.*" Continue by asserting, "*It's my intent to turn my organs of perception inward on the level of my public field of empathy.*" Next assert, "*It's my intent to fill my public field of empathy with prana and pure consciousness.*" Take a few moments to enjoy the shift. Then assert, "*It's my intent that healing energy and consciousness radiate from my public field of empathy into the area of my client's body I've chosen to heal.*" Don't do anything after that. The prana and consciousness emerging from your healing space will radiate into the body parts you have in mind.

Continue the healing for fifteen minutes. After fifteen minutes, visualize that the body part you chose to heal is glowing with radiant good health. Then recharge yourself. Once you're fully recharged, count from one to five. When you reach the number five, open your eyes. Give your client five more minutes to enjoy the effects of the healing. Then bring the client out of the exercise by having them open their eyes.

---

### Exercise: Healing Your Relationship to the Source of Healing

In this exercise, you will use your healing space to enhance your relationship to the source of healing. This will make you a more effective healer and will enhance your experience of transcendence. To begin the process, sit in a comfortable position with your back straight. Then close your eyes and breathe yogically for two to three minutes. Count backward from five to one and from ten to one. Then use the standard method to relax your muscles and to center yourself in your subtle field of energy and consciousness.

When you're ready to continue, assert, "*It's my intent to center myself in my transcendent field of empathy.*" Continue by asserting, "*It's my intent to turn my organs of perception inward on the level of my transcendent field of empathy.*" Continue by asserting, "*It's my intent that the source of healing radiates its healing energy and consciousness through my field of empathy into my body, soul, and spirit.*" Don't do anything after that. Just enjoy the process.

After fifteen minutes, count from one to five. When you reach the number five, open your eyes and bring yourself out of the exercise. Repeat as needed.

## Stroking and Laying On of Hands

Now that you've learned to use your healing space to heal yourself, another person, and your relationship to the source of healing, you're ready to use stroking in the laying on of hands. Stroking can be integrated into any session of laying on of hands. The best time to perform stroking is at the end of a session—after you've performed vibrational healing and empathetic healing. Stroking can be practiced in a number of ways, but no matter which way the hands are used, it is essential that you stay centered in your subtle field.

In the first part of stroking, you will make circular passes within your client's aura above the diseased area. To do that, you will lift your masculine hand from the surface of your client's body (keeping it within his or her etheric aura) while you hold your feminine hand at shoulder level with the palm up.

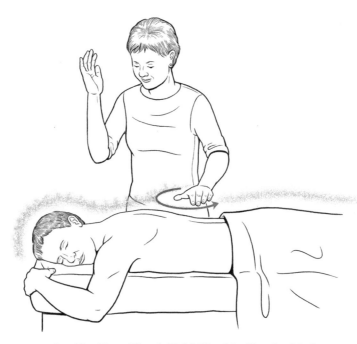

*Stroking Your Client's Field: Hand in Circular Motion*

Then you will begin making slow, circular hand motions about three inches (8 cm) above the diseased tissue with your positively charged hand. Keep your positive hand flat, with your palm down while circling the problem area. The circles should always be made in a clockwise direction. Your breathing (through the nose) should be slightly forced, as if under pressure. As you make the circular passes, pay attention to the palm of your hand and feel healing energy flowing rhythmically through it. Then begin making the motions more rapid while you feel healing energy flowing from your hand into your client's body. Feel it working its way into the diseased tissue, healing it completely. Continue with this variation until you feel satisfied the healing energy has had a positive effect.

After completing the circular passes, make a long fluid pass over the front of their body with your hands apart and fingers trailing, from their head to their feet. You'll probably have to stand up to do this. Hold your breath while you're making the pass, inhaling just as you begin at your client's head and exhaling after you've completed the pass at their feet.

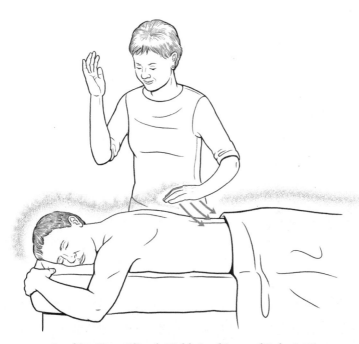

*Stroking Your Client's Field: Stroking and Polarization*

Make seven passes using the same technique. At the end of each pass, shake your hands away from your client in order to remove any negativity that you might have picked up as you made the pass through his or her aura. When you've completed the seven passes, you will count from one to five and bring yourself out of the healing. Then you will recharge yourself.

Let your client enjoy the healing energy while you recharge yourself. Then bring your client out of the exercise by counting from one to five and having him or her open their eyes. Take the next few minutes to get feedback from your client and to answer their questions. When your client is gone, rinse your hands with cold water to remove any residual negativity.

### Exercise: Self-Healing with Empathy and Vibration

In the exercise that follows, you will use empathetic healing and vibrational healing to heal yourself through laying on of hands. Once you've chosen the ailment you want to heal, find a comfortable position with your back straight. Then close your eyes and breathe yogically for two to three minutes. Count backward from five to one and from ten to one. Then use the standard method to relax your muscles and to center yourself in your subtle field of energy and consciousness.

When you're ready to continue, pay attention to the rhythms of your body and allow your bodily rhythms to direct the rhythm of your breathing. At most this should take two minutes. Once you've synchronized your internal rhythms with your breath, bring your attention to your hands. Your breath should be slightly forced, and you should continue breathing without separation between inhalation and exhalation until you feel your hands vibrate and get hot.

After a short time, your hands will become warm and begin to vibrate. This will quickly be replaced by a deep, almost overwhelming compassion for yourself. This will trigger the central pranic vibration, which will begin in the central cavity of your body. When the central pranic vibration reaches your hands and replaces the original vibration, place your hands on either side of the afflicted area (remember to keep them apart) and begin healing with vibration for the next five minutes. After five minutes, assert, *"It's my intent to center myself in my personal field of empathy."* Continue by asserting, *"It's my intent to turn my organs of perception inward on the level of my personal field of empathy."* Next, assert, *"It's my intent to fill my personal field of empathy with prana and pure consciousness."* Take a few moments to enjoy the shift. Then assert, *"It's my intent that healing energy and consciousness flows through my personal field of empathy into the area of my body I've chosen to heal."*

Keep your hands on either side of the afflicted area and continue the healing for five minutes more. Complete your work on the afflicted area by visualizing that the diseased tissue is perfectly healthy. Then remove your hands, count from one to five, and bring yourself out of the exercise. Repeat as needed.

---

### Exercise: Healing with Empathy, Vibration, and Stroking

In the exercise that follows, you will use vibrational healing, empathetic healing, and stroking to heal a physical ailment in another person's body.

Once you've explained what you will be doing and answered your client's questions, have him or her lie down on his or her back and breathe deeply through the nose. Find a comfortable position with your back straight. Then close your eyes and breathe deeply through the nose for two to three minutes. Count backward from five to one and from ten to one. Then use the standard method to relax your muscles and to center yourself in your subtle field of energy and consciousness.

When you're ready to continue, pay attention to the rhythms of your body and allow your bodily rhythms to direct the rhythm of your breathing. At most, this should take one or two minutes. Once you've synchronized your internal rhythms with your breath, bring your attention to your hands. Your breath should be slightly forced, and you should continue breathing without separation between inhalation and exhalation until you feel your hands vibrate and get hot.

After a short time, you should begin to feel a deep, almost overwhelming compassion for your client. This will trigger the central pranic vibration, which will begin in the central cavity of your body. When the central pranic vibration reaches your hands and replaces the original vibration, place your hands on your client's head—one on each side of the temple. Perform a general healing for about five minutes using prana healing (see chapter 4) and auric healing (see chapter 5) through the minor energy centers in your hands. Then place your hands on either side of the afflicted area and continue healing with vibration for two to three minutes.

When you're ready to continue, assert, "*It's my intent to center myself in the public field of empathy.*" Continue by asserting, "*It's my intent to turn my organs of perception inward on the level of the public field of empathy.*" Next, assert, "*It's my intent to fill my public field of empathy with prana and pure consciousness.*" Take a few moments to enjoy the shift. Then assert, "*It's my intent that healing energy and consciousness flows through my public field of empathy into the area of my client's body I've chosen to heal.*" Take another five minutes to heal with vibration and empathy.

Other healing techniques may spontaneously appear during the laying on of hands. They will not interfere with the healing, and I encourage you to use mental healing, chakra healing, and color healing along with vibrational healing and empathetic healing, especially when you're working on a particularly stubborn problem.

When you're finished working on the ailment, visualize that it is healthy and radiating prana freely. Then return to your client's head and place your hands on his or her temples, again with your hands opposite each other. Take a couple of minutes to fill your client's aura with rays of energy from your heart chakra and third eye. Feel your client absorb the energy through the skin and feel it recharging every cell in his or her body. Then visualize your client happy, healthy, and smiling radiantly. After five minutes, begin stroking your client's aura. Make circular strokes at your client's crown chakra. Then move downward until you've worked on all seven traditional chakras. Complete the process by making seven strokes down their body from their head to their feet.

When you've finished the last seven strokes, recharge yourself. Then return to normal consciousness by counting from one to five. When you reach the number five, open your eyes. Release your client as well. Have your client open his or her eyes and give you feedback. After the healing session, rinse your hands with cold water to remove any residual negativity.

## Summary

In this chapter, you learned how to achieve the central pranic vibration and to enhance your empathy so that you can become a more effective healer. You also learned to use your three fields of empathy to create a compassionate space where you can heal your clients. Afterward, you learned how to perform vibrational healing and empathetic healing, and to combine them with stroking to perform a complete session of the laying on of hands.

In the next chapter, I will answer some of the most common questions people have about spiritual healing. The answers are based on my experience and the experience of some of the great healers whose methods have been passed down to us through the ages.

# Chapter 11

# Questions and Answers about Healing

Over the years, I've been asked many questions about spiritual healing. I would like to answer some of the most common ones now. My answers to these questions are based on my own experience, not on any rigid doctrine or theology. They're subjective and, in the end, you must let your own intuition and conscience guide you.

## Multiple Healings

*Is it a good idea to work on more than one person during an absentee-healing session?*

The answer to this depends on the healer, the amount of time he or she has available for absentee healing, and his or her level of vitality. Vitality depends on several things: the healer's ability to surrender to the healing force, his or her ability to store prana, and, of course, the healer's state of mental, emotional, and physical health.

The only rule to follow is, "never strain yourself." If you feel that healing has become an effort or if you are exhausted or you feel a lack of vitality afterward, then you've worked on too many people during the same healing session. And you should cut down.

Most spiritual healers find that after they've been performing healings for a short time, their capacity increases and they're able to work with more clients for longer periods of time.

# The Healer's Reaction

*How should the healer feel after performing a healing session?*

The answer is fairly simple. If you remain detached by remaining centered in your subtle field during the healing, you will feel invigorated afterward.

By acting as a channel, you will benefit from the energy and consciousness that radiates through your subtle field. If you do several healings in a row, however, you might feel a mild dissipation, which is caused by an excessive expenditure of personal vitality.

With every healing, you expend a small amount of personal prana that must be differentiated from the healing energy (prana) that is being channeled through you during a healing session. This loss is inconsequential when you perform one or two healings. When you do several healings in a day, or more than one healing in a session, there can be a drain of personal prana. This drain will often be experienced as an unusual form of exhaustion that can make you feel lethargic and sleepy or nervous and cranky. Neither situation is dangerous if you naturally recharge yourself.

If you organize your schedule with this in mind, allowing ample time to rest, play, and sleep, by the next day you should be completely recharged and full of vitality.

# Resistant Clients

*Should a healer work on everyone*
*who comes to them for healing?*

As long as I get permission, I've always worked on anyone I intuitively felt would benefit from spiritual healing. This means I work on people who at first appear resistant, but in such cases I always explain that the healing may take time and may not be complete. My decisions have always been based on my intuition and then scrutinized by my conscience. When I get the okay from both, I begin and won't be put off by any difficulties or adverse conditions that present themselves later. It's important to remember that if you intuitively feel that it's appropriate to work with someone, there is a great likelihood your work will benefit him or her.

## The Length of a Healing Session

*How long should an absentee healing session last?*

There is no standard length of time for an absentee healing. I combine absentee healing with an introductory meditation, and the entire process takes about forty minutes. In a forty-minute meditation, I take about twenty minutes for the actual healing. This is an average. Sometimes I take more time and sometimes less, depending upon how I feel. In a laying on of hands session, I usually spend about thirty minutes doing the actual healing. Time itself is not the most important factor in healing. I've seen people healed instantaneously after being touched for just a few seconds.

## How Long Before the Client Is Healed?

*How long will it take to heal a physical ailment?*

The healer never knows for sure how long it will take to heal a particular ailment or even if the ailment can be completely healed. Healing is a process of transmutation. Although healing energy and consciousness are more powerful than the energy that supports disease, it may take time for the client's physical body to use what has been transferred by the healer.

It's also important to remember that in many cases healing the mind and the emotions is a prerequisite for healing a physical ailment. Although we aim for immediate results, it's unrealistic to expect an immediate physical healing when a client's soul and spirit still suffer from the effects of an unhealthy lifestyle and negative attachments.

It's not unusual for a healer to work for an extended time with a client before he or she achieves the desired result. I had such an experience with one of my earliest clients who suffered from a serious eye disorder. He was an eighty-two-year-old man who had lost his peripheral vision and was left with tunnel vision only. To compound matters, he suffered from hemorrhages in both eyes, which further distorted his vision. Neither of his conditions could be treated by orthodox medicine. We began working together twice a week. At first, I had to push through blockages to get healing energy to his eyes. Performing color healing was particularly difficult. His lack of receptivity also made visualization difficult. I intuitively knew it was appropriate to continue working with him, so I did. After the first month, things slowly began to change. The blockages began to fall away and little by little my visualizations became more vivid and protracted.

Six weeks into treatment, he went to see his eye doctor and he was told, to his amazement, that his vision had improved. He couldn't see the improvement at that point, but he was greatly encouraged.

We continued to work together with a renewed enthusiasm, and within one week he began to experience a change in his vision. First the improvement lasted only a few hours, but by the end of the seventh week of treatment, the improvement became more protracted and the distortion began to disappear. He went back to his doctor at the end of the eighth week and he was told there was a remarkable change in his condition. Not only had the distortion been corrected, so had the hemorrhages. We continued to work and the tunnel vision began to improve. For the first time in months, he began to read again, first with a magnifying glass, but a short time later without one. Between the sixth and tenth week of treatment, his doctor estimated he regained 80 percent of his sight.

## The Best Times for Healing

*When is the best time to perform healing?*

There isn't one answer that can be applied to all conditions and all circumstances. Each of us has a different lifestyle that must be taken into consideration. I recommend you work when you're relaxed and have nothing pressing on your mind. It's not a good idea to work when you're anxious or sleepy. I usually recommend that students of healing perform absentee healing in the early evening after they've completed their day's work. If your schedule permits, you can work in the morning as well.

# Picking Up Diseases

*Can the healer contract a disease from his clients?*

Excluding contagious diseases, it's unheard of for a healer to pick up any disease from his client that directly affects his physical body. However, in both the laying on of hands and absentee healing, the healer is making contact with his client on the subtle levels of energy and consciousness. Although there can't be any direct transfer of physical disease, it is possible for the healer to pick up distorted energy and consciousness that can manifest as negative feelings, emotions, and thoughts. There should be no problem if the healer remains detached by remaining centered in his or her strong center in the body and subtle field. However, if the healer's individual mind and ego inserts themselves into the healing process, there can be a problem. To mitigate it, practice Hara breathing and the standard method regularly until you can stay securely centered in your subtle field during the healing process.

# Dangerous Healing Techniques

*Healers can use different techniques to perform spiritual healing—how do I know when a technique that I use is counter-productive or potentially dangerous to my client and myself?*

While it's true that people from different healing traditions perform spiritual healing, not all the techniques they use are safe. Your safety and your client's safety must be your most important concern when you perform spiritual healing. You must refrain from doing anything that may endanger your client or yourself.

One principle that should never be ignored is this: it's never safe to push or pull energy through your subtle field or your client's subtle field during a healing session.

In some techniques currently used, healers pull energy and/or consciousness from the earth or from higher planes into their subtle field and then use them to perform spiritual healing. Pulling or pushing energy and/or consciousness through either your subtle field or your client's subtle field is dangerous for two reasons. First, there is no guarantee that the energy and/or consciousness you're pulling is pure and free of distorted fields. You may believe they're pure, but unless you are properly centered in the authentic mind (and subtle field) and your discernment is excellent and you can assess the differences between fields of energy and consciousness with universal qualities and those with individual qualities, there is no guarantee that the client will receive only healing energy and consciousness during the session.

The second principle is this: pulling or pushing energy and/or consciousness through a person's subtle field will weaken surface boundaries, including the surface boundaries surrounding chakra fields, auric fields, and resource fields. The surface boundaries of these fields are composed of luminescent fibers that crisscross each other in every conceivable direction. These fibers are designed to stretch as the field expands and to allow toxic energy and consciousness to be ejected. But they're not designed to allow large amounts of toxic energy and/or consciousness to pass through them regularly in both directions.

When energy and consciousness are pulled and pushed through them on a regular basis, surface boundaries begin to weaken and distorted fields begin to enter the subtle field with impunity. This can cause problems for both healer and client. Distorted fields can disrupt a healer's discernment and make it difficult or even impossible for him or her to perform spiritual healing. In time they can accumulate in the healer's subtle field and become the foundation of both karmic patterns and physical disease. For the client, the introduction of distorted fields— even in small amounts—can prevent a healing from taking place. In extreme cases, they can make the client's original condition worse.

## Summary

In this chapter, I answered some of the most common questions people have about spiritual healing. You learned to have patience because some healings take time, and you learned how to deal with resistant clients. You also learned that not all healing techniques are safe and that you must discriminate between those that are safe and reliable and those that are potentially dangerous. In the next chapter, you will learn to heal your soul by healing karmic patterns and energetic traumas.

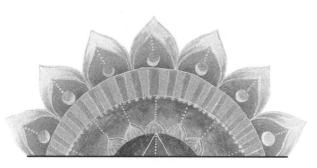

# Part 3

# Healing Your
# Soul and Spirit

# Chapter 12
# Healing Karmic Patterns

All human beings are born with the capacity to share pleasure, love, and intimacy with other people. Unfortunately, it's rare to find a person who can do this effortlessly. That's because most people alive today have karmic patterns that limit the radiating of consciousness and flow of prana through their subtle field on the level of soul. That makes it difficult for them to know themselves, to be themselves, and to express themselves freely.

To understand how karmic patterns can interfere with the healthy functions of your soul, it's essential to know how karma functions and how karmic baggage can create self-limiting patterns that affect your health and your relationships.

## What Is Karma?

The ancient Sanskrit word *karma* comes from the root *kri*, "to act," and it signifies an activity or action. In the West, karma has been defined as the cumulative effect of action. In a limited way, this is true, though the great religions of the East go beyond this definition by describing karma in terms of both its structure and function.

Jainism, an Indian spiritual tradition that stresses aestheticism, nonviolence, and reverence for life, views karma as an aggregate of subtle matter that accumulates in the human energy system and veils the consciousness of the self and everything that emerges from it. According to this ancient religion, karma has eight functional aspects: it obscures comprehension; it obscures awareness; it produces counterfeit feelings (emotions and sensations); it deludes a person (veils the truth); it is age-determining; it defines personality by creating behavioral patterns; it determines status and therefore psychic well-being; and it disrupts personal power. The first four aspects are obstructive; the remaining four are not (though they are self-limiting) since they obstruct the free radiation of consciousness and prana through the subtle field.

From what we've learned so far, it's clear that karma is far more complex than the abstract principle that guarantees that you will reap what you sow. Karma is a dynamic force of nature that manifests will and intent. Through its ability to create attachment, it defines a person and limits his or her freedom. Much like gravity, the polarity karma creates between the cause and its effect attracts a person to objects, fields of energy with individual qualities, and living beings (based on past actions) and then binds them by creating patterns of behavior that are self-limiting and often self-destructive.

## What Is Karmic Baggage?

Karmic baggage is composed of energy with individual qualities and the distorted consciousness that supports it. People carry both in their subtle field from one lifetime to another.

The distorted energy and consciousness I'm talking about create pressure and muscle aches when you're stressed and produce anxiety, self-doubt, and confusion when they're consciously or unconsciously activated. In fact, karmic baggage in one form or another is the principle source of both human suffering and physical disease.

When enough karmic baggage becomes trapped in the subtle field, it creates patterns that disrupt the free radiation of consciousness and prana. Since it's prana that sustains pleasure, love, intimacy, and healing, and it's consciousness that makes you aware of them all, any disruption in their ability to radiate freely through the subtle field will disrupt relationships and create a fertile environment for the development of disease.

The importance of pleasure, love, and intimacy as well as a continuous radiation of healing energy and consciousness in one's life cannot be overstated. The Yoga Sutras teach that negative sensations, feelings, emotions, and thoughts will flood through one's subtle field whenever the radiation of prana and healing consciousness have been restricted and/or pushed out of one's conscious awareness.

## Karmic Baggage on the Spiritual Level

Karmic baggage can become trapped and build up within the subtle field on any level. The more karmic baggage is trapped on a particular level, the more difficult it will be for consciousness and prana to radiate freely.

When an inordinate amount of karmic baggage has become trapped in one's subtle field on the spiritual level, one will find oneself trapped in self-limiting patterns that disrupt the activities and universal qualities that are within the domain of spirit. These include the qualities of good character as well as the activities that enhance pleasure, love, intimacy, and joy. Much like the proverbial dog chasing its tail, self-limiting patterns on the level of spirit will keep one busy with activities that lead nowhere and that merely serve to perpetuate the pattern. This fruitless merry-go-round, which is called the *Dance of Shiva* by tantric adepts, is ultimately self-defeating and antagonistic to self-awareness and freedom of self-expression. *Living in a spiritual desert* is a phrase often used to describe a person trapped in such a condition.

The accumulation of karmic baggage on the spiritual level can cause collateral problems in addition to those already mentioned. It can disrupt boundaries (particularly the surfaces of the auric fields). And it can disrupt the synchronistic functions of your vehicles of energy and consciousness on the level of spirit.

In time, as karmic baggage accumulates and usurps the functions of spirit, a person can fall prey to a counterfeit spirituality (supported by counterfeit spiritual experiences). A counterfeit spirituality is one that denies a person's eternal relationship with Universal Consciousness—the source of healing—and their state of enlightenment.

## Karmic Baggage on the Mental Level

An inordinate accumulation of karmic baggage on the level of mind that blocks the free radiation of consciousness and prana will disrupt awareness, creativity, peace of mind, memory, and the normal balance of inductive and deductive reasoning. In fact, once there has been a disruption in the transmission of prana on the mental level, one will find it almost impossible to go inward. Instead, one will find oneself trapped in the internal dialogue (the incessant chatter of the individual mind and ego) and reactive to fields of distorted energy and consciousness on the mental level.

The unfortunate individual who's had their mental functions disrupted by karmic baggage will often feel like their mind has become foggy or is racing out of control. In extreme situations, when enough distorted consciousness and energy has been introduced into a person's subtle field, on the mental level, patterns can develop that can be so compelling (badgering and nagging a person) with alien ideas, attitudes, and beliefs that the beleaguered individual can begin to think (and eventuality behave) in anti-self and/or antisocial ways.

## Karmic Baggage on the Emotional Level

Any disruption of healing consciousness and prana on the level of emotion, by karmic baggage, will restrict one's ability to express or even sense emotional energy.

There are only four authentic human emotions: anger, fear, pain, and joy. They're authentic because they emerge from the chakras deep within the world of soul. Anger emerges through the second chakra, fear through the third chakra, pain through the fourth chakra, and joy through the fifth chakra.

When healing consciousness and prana are flowing freely and are not restricted by karmic baggage and/or attachment on the emotional level, the four authentic emotions will be expressed spontaneously without fear and there will be a purging of the emotion through the facial musculature and the organs of expression—the mouth and the eyes.

Human beings have the ability to express these four emotions by crying, yelling, screaming, etc., as well as by expressing them through their eyes and facial musculature. When an emotion is expressed spontaneously and is resolved, there will be a feeling of satisfaction, which indicates that the pent-up emotional energy has been purged and a healthy flow of prana has been restored.

Karmic baggage, which blocks the flow of consciousness and prana on the emotional level, rarely allows emotions to reach the third or final stage of this process, called resolution. This leaves behind a residue of emotional energy that no amount of crying, screaming, or shouting will release. Emotional energy that has not been expressed spontaneously will become part of the karmic baggage that is deposited in the auric fields surrounding the body on the emotional level.

### Karmic Baggage on the Etheric Level

Feelings emerge from the etheric plane, which means they vibrate within a lower spectrum of frequencies than emotions, which emerge from the world of soul. Hence, feelings are less precise than emotions. The vibration of some feelings is so low that they closely resemble physical sensations. In fact, many of the most common psychosomatic ailments, which have been linked to physical stress, are etheric ailments caused by the accumulation of karmic baggage on the etheric level. Chronic fatigue syndrome, attention deficit disorder, chronic and acute depression, anxiety disorders, and panic attacks, as well as shortness of breath, back pain, and colitis, are some of the more well-known ailments that are caused by the inordinate accumulation of karmic baggage on the etheric level.

Intuition, which most people experience as a gut feeling or vague perception of the truth, emerges into conscious awareness on the etheric level. If the buildup of karmic baggage is too great, it can inhibit one's intuitive awareness; that in turn can make it increasingly difficult to accept the validity of one's perceptions and to make decisions that are appropriate and enhance one's life and relationships.

### Karmic Baggage on the Physical Level

Sensations and physical pleasure emerge from the physical level, which means they vibrate in a lower spectrum of frequencies than feelings. When the free radiation of consciousness and prana on the physical level has been disrupted by karmic baggage, physical sensations and physical pleasure will be disrupted as well. This can result in sexual dysfunction, which includes impotence and premature ejaculation in men and orgasmic dysfunction in women. In fact, almost any type of aversion to normal sexual stimulation and pleasure can be traced back to the same root cause, a disruption in the free radiation of consciousness and prana on the physical level.

Since karmic baggage on the physical level can have a negative impact on stamina and strength, it can also have a disruptive effect on physical performance. By accumulating at strategic points in the physical body, karmic baggage can compel a person to compensate for added density on the physical level by making micro-movements that strain the body at its weakest points (the joints and points where tendons and cartilage meet). This added stress, particularly for athletes who demand top performance from their physical body, can cause serious injury.

When karmic baggage becomes too great a burden, it can disrupt the production of pleasure-producing compounds in the brain. The disruption of body chemistry can then lead to physical dependency, particularly if the afflicted person is unable to control themselves and their immediate environment.

From our study of karma and karmic baggage, it should be clear that to heal your soul it's essential to release the karmic baggage that disrupts the free radiation of consciousness and prana through your subtle field, which is responsible for disrupting your health and your relationships. The first step will be to learn to scan your auric fields for karmic baggage.

## Scanning for Karmic Baggage

Although scanning for karmic baggage is essentially the same technique as remote viewing, there are a few differences that must be taken into account. When scanning for karmic baggage, you will be using your intent and mental attention for the sole purpose of discerning the energetic condition of your subtle field—in particular the auric fields. That's because in healing the soul it's the distorted energy deposited in a person's auric fields that is most important—not the effect it can have on the condition of the client's physical body. Of course, rightness and wrongness play an important part in your scan the same way they do in remote viewing. They point to areas of the subtle field that contain distorted energy.

---

### Exercise: Scanning for Karmic Baggage

To begin scanning your subtle field for karmic baggage, find a comfortable position with your back straight. Close your eyes and breathe yogically for two to three minutes. Then count backward from five to one and ten to one. Use the standard method to relax your muscles and center yourself in your subtle field of energy and consciousness. Then assert, "*It's my intent to create a visual screen eight feet (2.5 m) in front of me.*" Once the visual screen appears, assert, "*It's my intent to visualize an image of myself on my visual screen.*"

Once the image appears, begin to scan the area between your physical body and the surface of your aura, which extends about eight feet (2.5 m) from the surface of your body space. Scan the front of your aura, the back, the sides, and even the areas on top of your head and below the bottom of your feet. Since the most disruptive karmic baggage will be stuck closest to your body, pay particular attention to the area that extends from the surface of your body to a distance of approximately two feet (0.5 m).

When you locate a field of karmic baggage, you will recognize it because its individual qualities—size, shape, density etc.—will stand out from the background of prana and pure consciousness in your subtle field. Continue to scan its entire length and record the information on its location, state, size, shape, density, polarity, level of activity, and surface texture. If information about its awareness, attitude, and personality emerges, record it as well. When you're satisfied with your scan and the information you've gathered, release the image of yourself and the visual screen. Then count from one to five. When you reach the number five, open your eyes. You will feel wide awake, perfectly relaxed, and better than you did before.

Before we move on, it's important to note that there is more than one way to locate karmic baggage. You can scan your auric field to locate a concentration of distorted energy like you just did or you can choose a pattern you want to release and use your intent to program your mental attention to locate the karmic baggage that supports it.

---

### Exercise: Releasing Karmic Baggage

Now that you've scanned your subtle field for karmic baggage, you're ready to heal a karmic pattern. To do that, you will use the prana box. Before you begin, choose a karmic pattern you want to heal. It could be anything that limits your personal power or your ability to share pleasure, love, intimacy, and joy. Self-sabotage is one such pattern, and so are feelings of insecurity or dependency.

After you've chosen a karmic pattern to heal, find a comfortable position with your back straight. Then close your eyes and breathe yogically for two to three minutes. Count backward from five to one and from ten to one. Then use the standard method to relax your muscles and to center yourself in your subtle field of energy and consciousness. Next, perform the orgasmic bliss mudra.

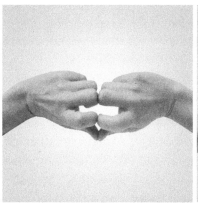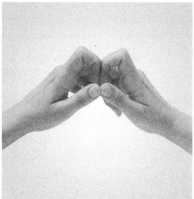

*The Orgasmic Bliss Mudra*

Hold the mudra while you assert, *"It's my intent to create a visual screen eight feet (2.5 m) in front of me."* Continue by asserting, *"It's my intent to visualize an image of myself on the visual screen."* Next, assert, *"It's my intent to see and feel the karmic baggage that provides the most support to the karmic pattern I've chosen to heal."* Once it appears, take a moment to scan it for size, shape, density, and level of activity. Then assert, *"It's my intent to create a prana box that surrounds the karmic baggage I've just experienced."*

Once you can see and/or sense the prana box, assert, *"It's my intent to fill the prana box with bliss."* Then assert, *"It's my intent that bliss releases the karmic baggage in my prana box."* Once the karmic baggage has been released, release the prana box. Then release the image of yourself on the visual screen. Release the screen. Then count from one to five and bring yourself out of the healing exercise.

Although it's possible to release a karmic pattern in one healing session, in some cases a karmic pattern is so complex that it has more than one field of karmic baggage that supports it. When you work on karmic patterns such as these, you will have to repeat the exercise you just performed on each field of karmic baggage in order to overcome the pattern completely.

Releasing karmic baggage is an important part of healing your soul. Another part that is often overlooked is healing energetic traumas that have disrupted the functions of soul.

## Trauma, the Inside Story

Although medical and mental health practitioners have studied the various forms of trauma for years, they still have trouble defining them. That's because it's almost impossible to define or even describe a traumatic event without taking into consideration the violence done to the survivor's subtle field of energy and consciousness. There is a simple reason for this: it's the violence done to the subtle field that is responsible for the most acute and enduring symptoms the survivor must endure.

To understand why a traumatic event can have a long-term effect on a person, it's important to recognize that every traumatic event is really a dual event that includes two traumas—a physical-psychological trauma and a subtle energetic trauma that is non-physical but no less real.

Memory of the physical and psychological trauma may be repressed, but the energetic trauma will continue to emerge into the survivor's consciousness for years as a disruption of authentic identity, motivation, and concentration as well as a disruption of their ability to express themselves freely. It will also contribute to the breakdown of the survivor's trust, which will disrupt self-esteem and make it difficult for the survivor to participate in long-term, intimate relationships.

All traumatic events, including past-life trauma, physical and psychological trauma, sexual trauma, and the trauma of neglect, have three things in common. They're all accompanied by a violent intrusion of distorted energy into the survivor's subtle field. The violence of the energetic intrusion will cause one or more energetic vehicles to be ejected. This is known as "fragmentation." And, the intrusion will disrupt the flow of prana though the survivor's subtle energy system. It's these three energetic effects that create lifelong problems for the survivor—problems that cannot normally be corrected with conventional therapy or orthodox medicine.

Since it's the intrusion of distorted energy into the survivor's subtle energy field that is responsible for all subsequent symptoms, you will learn to heal intrusions first.

## Intrusions

An intrusion is created by the violent projection of distorted energy into a person's subtle field. If you're the target of an intrusion, you may feel like a pin or a dart has punctured your skin when it makes contact with your subtle field. The intrusion may also make you feel like you're being smothered or like a wave of discordant energy is pouring into you.

You don't have to be in physical contact with the perpetrator to be the target of an intrusion. People who are attached to distorted fields of energy can project them into your subtle field when they think about you, have strong feelings about you, or have the desire to change, manipulate, control, or punish you.

Many survivors make matters worse by accepting the intrusion as a function of their own soul. If you're a target of a projection of distorted energy and you become the thinker of the thought or you invest your personal will, desire, and/or intent in the idea, emotion, feeling, or sensation that emerges from the distorted field, you will become attached to it. Once you're attached to the intrusion, it's just a matter of time before it becomes trapped in your subtle field and integrated into your soul as well as the corresponding functions of your individual mind and ego.

Below are some guidelines that will help you to determine which thoughts, ideas, emotions, feelings, and sensations are generated by your own mind and which have entered your subtle field as intrusion of distorted energy.

### Symptoms of Intrusions

1. The introduction of disturbing thoughts, ideas, and feelings that are out of the context of what you're doing or press on you from the outside are caused by intrusions.

2. Sudden weakness, confusion, or anxiety about what you want and/or need are all caused by intrusions.

3. The appearance of thoughts, feelings, and sensations that try to manipulate, change, or control what you want or do, or that dwell on your defects—especially those you cannot change—are caused by intrusions.

4. A personality change that has made you feel fragile or overly reactive to other people and the energy they project is caused by an intrusion.

5. Fear of large groups accompanied by feelings of vulnerability can be caused by intrusions.

6. A shift in your sense of self that makes you feel self-conscious and/or insecure is caused by an intrusion.

7. Both alienation from your body and/or physical numbness are caused by intrusions.

8. The sudden feeling that you're being smothered by the needs and expectations of another person is caused by an intrusion.

9. Feelings of exhaustion and/or the feeling that you're being drained by people at least some of the time are caused by intrusions.

10. The inability to express your true feelings and/or ideas can be caused by intrusions.

Our list is only a sample. But if you feel trapped by any persistent issue or pattern that continuously interferes with your ability to manifest a strong, life-affirming identity or you know a person who has interfered with your ability to be yourself or to express yourself freely, then it's likely that your subtle field has been penetrated by an intrusion, even if you can't associate your symptoms with a specific event.

---

## Exercise: Releasing Intrusions

Releasing an intrusion is a relatively simple process. Before you begin, choose a feeling, attitude, blockage, or self-limiting pattern that creates an irrational fear of a particular person, place, or thing. You can also choose a feeling or pattern that consistently interferes with your ability to be yourself, express yourself freely, and/or achieve your goals (use the above list as a guide).

Examples of feelings caused by intrusions are panic, foreboding, rage, frustration, anxiety, alienation, arrogance, contempt, chronic irritation, and annoyance. Examples of patterns caused by intrusions include self-doubt, self-sabotage, helplessness, despondency, dependency, insecurity, indolence, and a lack of self-worth.

Once you've chosen a pattern or feeling to work on, find a comfortable position with your back straight. Then close your eyes and breathe deeply through your nose for two to three minutes. Use the standard method to relax your muscles and to center yourself in your subtle field of energy and consciousness. Then perform the orgasmic bliss mudra.

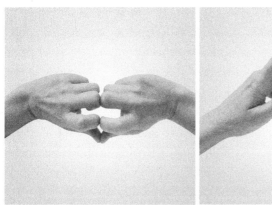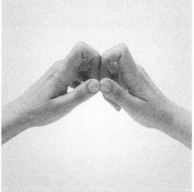

*The Orgasmic Bliss Mudra*

Continue to hold it while you assert, "*It's my intent to locate the intrusion in my subtle energy field that is most responsible for causing the* (feeling or pattern here) *I've chosen to release.*" Then assert, "*It's my intent to create a prana box that surrounds the intrusion.*" Once you can see and/or sense the prana box, continue by asserting, *"It's my intent to fill the prana box I cre-ated with bliss."* Then assert, *"It's my intent that bliss releases the intrusion in my prana box."*

As soon as the intrusion has been released, there will be a sense of relief that is often accompanied by a pop that indicates that the only thing that remains in your prana box is bliss. Once you've released the intrusion, release the prana box. Then re-lease the orgasmic bliss mudra. Take ten minutes to enjoy the changes you experience. Then count from one to five and bring yourself out of the meditation.

Like patterns created by karmic baggage, some patterns cre-ated by intrusions are so complex that you will have to repeat the exercise on each intrusion in order to overcome the symp-toms of the trauma completely.

## Fragmentation

Your subtle field will become fragmented whenever an energetic ve-hicle has been ejected from it. The most common cause of fragmenta-tion is a traumatic event caused by the intrusion of distorted energy in your subtle field. Fragmentation can take place on any level at any time during any phase of a person's life, including the nine months between conception and birth.

Fragmentation and its collateral effects have become so common that healing them by decontaminating and reintegrating energetic vehicles has become an essential part of karmic healing and energy work. That's because energetic vehicles carry out a host of vital func-tions. They allow you to form an authentic identity and to interact with your environment on both the physical and non-physical levels. Energetic vehicles also help you to manifest your soul urge and par-ticipate in intimate relationships.

To heal fragmentation, you must first release the intrusions that pushed an energetic vehicle out of your body space. Once those intru-sions have been released, you must locate the energetic vehicle that has been ejected. Then you must decontaminate it and reintegrate it into your subtle field. To locate an energetic vehicle that has been ejected from your subtle field and decontaminate it, you will use the same technique used to locate and release karmic baggage.

Once you've located and decontaminated an energetic vehicle, you must reintegrate it so that it's congruent. For an energetic vehicle to be congruent, it must be centered exactly in the middle of your body space. Congruence is important for several reasons. It permits the re-integrated vehicle to function synchronistically with other energetic vehicles in your subtle field. It facilitates the uninterrupted flow of prana through it. And it allows you to reintegrate it into your authentic identity.

### Exercise: Healing Fragmentation

To heal fragmentation, find a comfortable position with your back straight. Then close your eyes and breathe yogically for two to three minutes. Use the standard method to relax your muscles and to center yourself in your subtle field of energy and consciousness. Then perform the orgasmic bliss mudra and hold it.

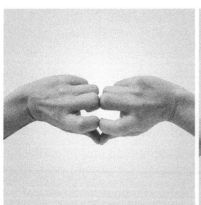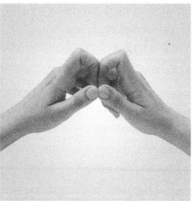

*The Orgasmic Bliss Mudra*

Next, assert, "*It's my intent to create a prana box around my energetic vehicle that has been ejected furthest from body space by the intrusion I released in the last exercise.*" Continue by asserting, "*It's my intent to fill the prana box I just created with bliss and to release all distorted energy in the energetic vehicle contained within it.*" Then assert, "*It's my intent to reintegrate the energetic vehicle within the prana box into my subtle field so that it's congruent.*" Don't do anything after that.

Your energetic vehicle will be decontaminated and reintegrated automatically. After the energetic vehicle has become congruent, take ten minutes to enjoy the effects. Then release the prana box, the orgasmic bliss mudra, and bring yourself out of the meditation by counting from one to five. Once congruence has been achieved, you will experience a sense of satisfaction, greater inner strength, and stability.

Since a traumatic experience can cause more than one energetic vehicle to be ejected, you may have to repeat the process more than once. To do that, always reintegrate the energetic vehicle that is farthest from your energy field first. In this way, you will consistently reintegrate all the energetic vehicles that were ejected by a traumatic experience.

Mistakes are inevitable. This means that you may reintegrate an energetic vehicle that still contains contaminants. If you do, symptoms will emerge almost immediately. The most common symptoms will be sudden anti-self and antisocial feelings that emerge from contaminants within the energetic vehicle. To correct the situation, you will have to remove the contaminants while the energetic vehicle is in your subtle field.

The technique is essentially the same one you used to heal fragmentation. Simply use your intent and mental attention to place the energetic vehicle in a prana box. Perform the orgasmic bliss mudra and hold it while you assert, "*It's my intent that bliss fills the prana box I just created and that it releases all the contaminants within it.*" Bliss will release any residual contamination, and it will also ensure that the energetic vehicle is properly integrated.

## Restoring the Flow of Prana

Whenever you experience a traumatic event, the flow of prana through your subtle field will be disrupted. The energetic flow will be partially restored once you've removed the intrusions and reintegrated your energetic vehicles that have been ejected. However, to fully restore the flow of prana to healthy levels, you must reactivate your thirteen chakras in body space as well as the first six chakras above it. The first six chakras above body space are located directly above your head. You can reactive these chakras by performing the exercise below.

---

### Exercise: Activating the Chakras in Body Space and Above It

To restore the flow of prana through your energy field, find a comfortable position with your back straight. Then close your eyes and breathe deeply through your nose for two to three minutes. When you're ready to continue, count backward from five to one then ten to one. Use the standard method to relax your muscles and to center yourself in your subtle field of energy and consciousness. Then assert, *"It's my intent to activate my first chakra."* Next assert, *"It's my intent to center myself in my first chakra field."* Continue in the same way by activating your second, third, fourth, fifth, sixth, and seventh chakras and by centering yourself in the corresponding chakra fields.

Take a few moments to enjoy the effects. Then activate your upper and lower etheric chakras, your upper and lower physical chakras, and your upper and lower physical-material chakras. Continue by centering yourself in their corresponding chakra fields. Once you've reactivated the chakras in body space, continue by reactivating your eighth, ninth, tenth, eleventh, twelfth, and thirteenth chakras located above your head. Then center yourself in their corresponding chakra fields. After you've activated all thirteen chakras in body space as well as the first six chakras above body space and centered yourself in their corresponding chakra fields, assert, *"On the levels of my first through thirteenth chakras, and the first six chakras above body space, it's my intent to turn my organs of perception inward."* Finally, assert, *"It's my intent to fill my thirteen chakra fields in my body space and the first six chakra fields above body space with prana."*

Take fifteen minutes to enjoy the changes you experience. Then count from one to five. When you reach the number five, open your eyes. You will feel wide awake, perfectly relaxed, and better than you did before.

By practicing this exercise for at least five days after you've released intrusions and reintegrated fragmented energetic vehicles, you will restore the flow of prana through your most important chakras and chakra fields. This will enable you to overcome many of the residual effects that are the legacy of the traumatic event you experienced.

## Summary

In this chapter, you learned how karmic baggage and energetic traumas can disrupt the functions of your soul. Then you learned how to release karmic baggage and to heal the energetic wounds caused by a traumatic event. You did that by releasing fields of karmic baggage intrusions, by restoring energetic vehicles to congruence, and by restoring the flow of prana through your subtle field.

It's important to note that not all intrusions cause fragmentation. Weaker intrusions are less disruptive. But they can create negative feelings, emotions, and attitudes. These intrusions can also be released using the technique you learned in this chapter. By releasing them, you will restore and maintain a strong sense of self, and you will enhance the wellness of both your body and soul.

In the next chapter, you will learn how to restore your soul to a condition of radiant good health by taking control of your seven polar fields and by enhancing the flow of prana through the three ruling meridians in Trishira.

# Chapter 13
# Restoring Your Soul

All people are burdened by karmic baggage and/or intrusions that have become trapped in their subtle field. The primary reason for this is not the density of the karmic baggage or the violence of the intrusions, it's a person's inability to occupy all their personal space.

Personal space includes the space occupied by the physical and subtle bodies. Most subtle bodies are the same size as your physical body, but some extend a few inches beyond their borders. The auric fields that surround them extend, on average, an additional twenty-six feet (8 m).

When you don't occupy all of your personal space, you lose power and control over your subtle field and subtle energy system. You can begin to remedy this problem by finding your strong center in your body and subtle energy field (see chapter 2) and by learning to fill your auric fields with prana (see chapter 5). But taking control of your personal space is not complete until you've taken control of it on all seven polar fields.

## The Seven Polar Fields

The first polar field is traditionally considered masculine in relationship to Atman, which means that, when you become masculine, you will radiate energy forward and you will become assertive. Energy fields that are inordinately masculine can create violent emotions and feelings. Some excessively masculine fields make it difficult for other energy fields that interact with them to maintain their position without being forced to contract or to become more receptive or feminine. In human interactions, the more masculine an energy field, the more assertive and controlling it can be and the more difficult it can be for people to maintain their sense of self without a struggle.

*Universal Consciousness*
*Atman*

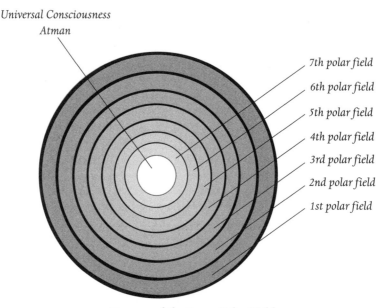

7th polar field
6th polar field
5th polar field
4th polar field
3rd polar field
2nd polar field
1st polar field

**Atman and the Seven Polar Fields**

The second polar field is traditionally considered feminine. When femininity becomes dominant in your subtle field, you will draw energy inward toward Atman and you will manifest power passively by being receptive.

Fields that are inordinately feminine can be extremely coercive, manipulative, and/or seductive. Becoming excessively feminine can make it difficult for energy fields around you to maintain their position because they can be pulled toward you. Coming in contact with an inordinately feminine field can disrupt your ability to express yourself freely and make it difficult for you to stay centered in your subtle field.

The third polar field is neuter or neutral, which means that it will not react to other energy fields within its environment. By remaining centered in the third polar field, you can remain undisturbed for long periods. That will enhance your ability to remain calm while you interact with energy fields that may be highly polarized. It will also enhance your ability to meditate and discern external fields of energy that interact with your subtle field.

When you're centered in the fourth polar field, energy with higher frequencies will become dominant and will move inward at the expense of energy with lower frequencies. Your identity will reflect this shift and you will be able to live with greater integrity. Functioning consciously through your fourth polar field will keep you centered in your subtle field even when you come into contact with highly polarized fields of energy with individual qualities. It will also prevent the individual mind and ego from gaining control over your subtle field and expressing their desire, will, and intent at your expense.

In the fifth polar field, interactions with other energy fields are a function of vibration, not movement, and are uniquely feminine. As you become more conscious of the fifth polar field and learn to function through it, your receptivity to the universal feminine will increase. As you embrace the universal feminine and her energy, you will experience more pleasure, love, intimacy, and joy.

In the sixth polar field, energetic interactions are a function of vibration, not movement, and are uniquely masculine. As you become more conscious of the sixth polar field and learn to function through it consciously, your receptivity to the universal masculine will be enhanced. As you embrace the universal masculine, your awareness will increase along with your discernment. This will enable you to manifest more personal power and give you more control over your subtle field.

In the seventh polar field, polarity is no longer defined by movement or vibration. In fact, Universal Consciousness emerges first into the phenomenal universe through the seventh polar field. From there, it descends through your subtle field from the fields of highest vibration to the fields of lowest vibration. Although this may appear to be a directional movement, it cannot be because time and space, as we experience them in a dualistic universe, do not exist within Universal Consciousness.

As you become conscious of the seventh polar field and begin to function through it consciously, you will recognize that your authentic mind is your true vehicle of awareness and self-expression. As Universal Consciousness radiates through your subtle field, without interference, you will experience *Sat Chit Ananda*, which is Sanskrit means "eternal life, all knowledge, and bliss."

## The Multidimensional Universe

Physics in the twenty-first century has validated what healers have known for centuries, namely that we live in a multidimensional universe that is more complex and exotic than most people believe. Physicists have had to expand their view of the universe to include non-physical dimensions that support the idea that the physical universe and quanta can be in more than one place at a time. It will also be necessary for you to expand your view of polarity from two polar fields—yin-yang, assertive-receptive, etc.—to seven polar fields through which consciousness and energy can emerge and through which human interactions take place.

In fact, as you become more conscious, you will see that polar relationships based on a bipolar universe exist only when you identify yourself as an individual being, separate from Universal Consciousness and the rest of the ecology of life in the universe of physical and subtle dimensions.

Unfortunately, your organs of perception (eyes, ears, nose, etc.) support the bipolar view of the universe. That's why it's so convincing. However, once you've made the transition to the authentic mind—and begun to center yourself in your subtle field—you will begin to experience the seven polar fields because your mind will not suffer the limitations imposed on it by either your organs of perception or the individual mind and ego.

By interacting consciously through the seven polar fields rather than two, you will be able to consciously experience seven different types of polar interactions with other subtle fields and living beings. And, you will be able to restore full control over your subtle field.

The polar field that dominates you at any particular time will determine how you interact energetically as well as the direction that subtle energy moves in relationship to Atman, the point where bliss enters your energy field.

In Sanskrit, *Atman* means "that which cannot be doubled." Atman emerges from the right side of your chest, directly across from the human heart and to the right of your heart chakra. You can think of it as the doorway through which Universal Consciousness enters your subtle field.

---

### Exercise: Healing a Polar Field

Now that you've learned how your seven polar fields function, you're ready to restore your control over a polar field on the levels of energy and consciousness. To do that, you will perform a meditation designed specifically for that purpose. In the meditation, you will begin by centering yourself in a specific polar field. Then you will perform the orgasmic bliss mudra and fill the polar field with bliss and prana. You will practice the exercise on your first polar field, which is masculine. Afterward, you can use the same technique to reassert control over your other six polar fields.

To begin the exercise, find a comfortable position with your back straight. Then close your eyes and breathe yogically for two to three minutes. Continue by counting backward from five to one and then ten to one. Use the standard method to relax the muscles of your physical body and to center yourself in your subtle field of energy and consciousness. Take a few moments to enjoy the shift. Then assert, "*It's my intent to center myself in my subtle field, in the first polar field.*" Continue by asserting, "*It's my intent to turn my organs of perception inward, in my subtle field, on the level of my first polar field.*" Immediately, your orientation will shift. And from your new vantage point, you will experience the awareness, emotions, and feelings associated with the first polar field. Continue by asserting, "*It's my intent to fill my subtle field, on the level of my first polar field, with prana.*" Then perform the orgasmic bliss mudra.

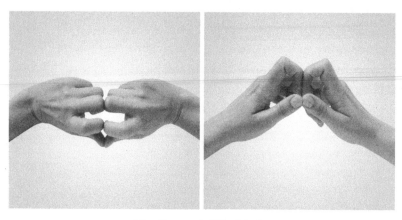

*The Orgasmic Bliss Mudra*

Hold the mudra while you assert, *"It's my intent to fill my subtle field, on the level of my first polar field, with pure consciousness."* Hold the mudra for another five minutes. Then release it and enjoy the changes you experience. After ten minutes, count from one to five and bring yourself out of the meditation.

To restore your control over all your polar fields, practice the same meditation on your second polar field the next day, and so on until, after seven days, you've performed the polar field meditation on all seven polar fields.

By practicing the seven meditations as a one-week cycle you will find it easier to remain centered in your subtle field in all seven polar fields. Taking back control of your subtle field on the level of soul will enable you to share your functions of soul freely with the people you love.

## Trishira and the Empowered Soul

Now that you've learned to take control of your subtle field in all seven polar fields, you're ready to take the next step, which is to empower yourself on the level of soul. To do that, you will enhance the flow of prana through the Ida, the Pingala, and the Sushumna (Governor). These three meridians are known as Trishira. In Sanskrit, *tri* means "three" and *shira* means "that which carries."

In chapter 6, you learned that meridians are streams of energy that connect chakras to one another and transmit prana through the human energy system. There are thousands of meridians, large and small, but just ten ruling meridians. Among these ten, the three most important are the Ida, the Pingala, and the Sushumna.

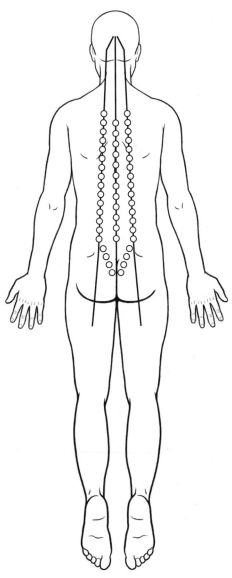

*The Meridians of Trishira*

### The Ruling Meridians

The Sushumna meridian originates at a position in your body that corresponds to the first chakra. Then it passes through the masculine pole (in the back) of the seven traditional chakras on its way up to the crown. The Ida and Pingala originate on either side of the first chakra. The Ida works its way up the left side of the Sushumna and passes through the left nostril. The Pingala works its way up the right side of the Sushumna and passes through the right nostril. Both the Ida and Pingala join the Sushumna again in the region of the sixth chakra.

The energy that radiates through Trishira has its origin at the base of the spine in the coiled serpent energy. The coiled serpent energy, also known as the Kundalini Shakti, is the most powerful manifestation of healing energy in your subtle field. Many of the practices of yoga and tantra are aimed at strengthening and balancing these three currents of energy. Indeed, both traditions teach that once the Kundalini Shakti has risen to the crown chakra, the Sushumna, Ida, and Pingala will merge into one massive channel of prana. When that happens, your entire field will become a celebration of the universe's healing and restorative power.

Raising the Kundalini Shakti to the crown chakra and beyond is a process that takes time, but by strengthening and balancing the flow of prana through the three meridians that make up Trishira, you can empower your soul and manifest more of its innate functions through your life and relationships.

Empowering your soul is a three-part process. First you must enhance the pressure in your subtle energy system by activating your first and seventh chakras. Then you must perform the Trishira Mudra (described below) while you stay centered in your subtle energy field. And finally, you must stimulate the minor energy centers along the three meridians that make up Trishira.

### The Energy Centers in Trishira

There are twelve minor energy centers along the Sushumna and twenty minor energy centers along the Ida. Twenty more energy centers are located along the Pingala in positions that correspond to the energy centers in the Ida. You will have to activate all of these energy centers in order to empower your soul.

Although this sounds like a big job, it won't be as difficult as you might imagine, because you will use your intent to activate the minor energy centers the same way you activated your chakras.

The energy centers along the Sushumna are located between major vertebrae. The energy centers in the Ida and Pingala are located in corresponding positions along the length of the two meridians.

You will activate the energy centers along the Sushumna first. Then you will activate the energy centers along the Ida. Finally, you will activate the energy centers along the Pingala.

In the next exercise, called the *Trishira meditation*, you will activate your first and seventh chakras. Then you will perform the *Trishira mudra* and, while you hold the mudra, you will use your intent to activate the minor energy centers in Trishira.

---

## Exercise: The Trishira Meditation

To begin the Trishira meditation, find a comfortable position with your back straight. Breathe yogically for two to three minutes. Then count from five to one, then from ten to one. Use the standard method to relax the muscles and to center yourself in your subtle field of energy and consciousness. Then assert, "*It's my intent to activate my first chakra.*" Continue by asserting, "*It's my intent to activate my seventh chakra.*" Take two to three minutes to enjoy the effects. After you've enjoyed the effects for two to three minutes you're ready to perform the Trishira mudra.

---

## Exercise: The Trishira Mudra

To perform the Trishira mudra, open your eyes and keep them slightly unfocused. Then slide your tongue past your lower teeth until the tip comes to rest at the lowest point. Put the tips of your corresponding fingers together so that your hands form a triangle. Then put the soles of your feet together so that they form another triangle. Continue to hold the mudra while you activate the minor energy centers along the Sushumna, Ida, and Pingala.

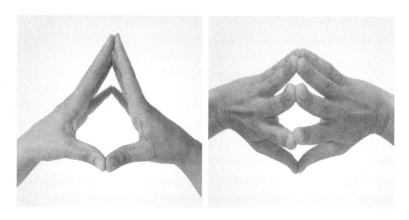

*The Trishira Mudra*

To activate the energy centers along the Sushumna, close your eyes again. Then assert, "*It's my intent to activate the energy centers along the Sushumna that belong to Trishira.*" Take a moment to enjoy the shift. Then assert, "*It's my intent to activate the energy centers along the Ida that belong to Trishira.*" Finally, assert, "*It's my intent to activate the energy centers along the Pingala that belong to Trishira.*" Continue to perform the Trishira mudra for ten more minutes more while you enjoy the enhanced flow of energy through the Sushumna, Ida, and Pingala. After five minutes, release the mudra, count from one to five, and open your eyes.

When you open your eyes, you will feel wide awake, perfectly relaxed, and better than you did before. Practice the exercise every day for two weeks and you will experience the profound benefits that come from restoring your soul.

# Summary

In this chapter, you learned to take back control of your seven polar fields. This will safeguard you against intrusions in the future that could disrupt your health on the level of soul. You also learned to restore your soul by performing the Trishira meditation.

In the next chapter, you will learn to do three things that will dramatically enhance the health of your spirit. You will learn to enhance the universal qualities associated with good character. You will learn to enhance your experience of inner peace by performing the *inner peace mudra*. And you will learn to center yourself in Atman, the doorway through which Universal Consciousness enters your field of spirit.

# Chapter 14
# Healing Your Spirit

Complete healing isn't possible without healing your spirit and liberating it from attachments and blockages. When asked about the importance of a liberated spirit, Meher Baba, one of India's most acclaimed spiritual teachers, said:

> *All life is an effort to attain freedom from self-created entanglement; it is a desperate struggle to undo what has been done under ignorance, to throw away the accumulated burden of the past—to find rescue from the debris left by a series of temporary achievements and failures.*[19]

It may come as a surprise to learn that freedom of this sort isn't reserved for Eastern adepts and masters alone. The truth is that spiritual freedom is available to everyone who has the yearning for it and who seeks it with integrity. That's because every human is an interdimensional being who has access to all the consciousness and healing energy he or she needs to heal his or her spirit and to experience spiritual freedom.

In order to heal your spirit and experience spiritual freedom, you must take control of your spirit and then empower it. You will begin that process by enhancing the universal qualities of good character.

---

19. Meher Baba, *Gems from the Discourses by Meher Baba* (New York: Circle Productions, 1945).

The qualities of good character include discipline, courage, perseverance, patience, long-suffering (the ability to endure during difficult times), and, most important of all, non-harming.

Everyone has these qualities in abundance, but not everyone can manifest them freely. That's because the functions of your spirit can be disrupted by attachments and blockages in your fields of energy and consciousness. To restore your spirit and to experience the benefits of good character, you will first learn more about these qualities and how they can be blocked. Then you will learn to use the skills you already have to enhance each universal quality associated with good character.

## The Essentials of Good Character

We will look at the qualities of good character in this order: discipline, courage, perseverance, patience, long-suffering, and non-harming.

*Discipline* is the ability to stay centered in your authentic mind—your true vehicle of consciousness—and to be yourself no matter how stressful your internal and/or external environment has become.

*Courage* is the willingness to defend your personal space on all levels of body, soul, and spirit, even when there is internal opposition from karmic baggage or external opposition from family, friends, or the institutions of your society.

*Perseverance* will emerge without restrictions of any sort once you're committed to sharing pleasure, love, intimacy, and joy no matter how stressful your internal and/or external environment may become.

*Patience* is the ability to stay centered in your authentic mind and subtle field even when projections of distorted energy interfere with your ability to express yourself and interact with other people.

*Long-suffering* is the ability to move forward or persevere in activities that are appropriate even when you must pay a price in personal well-being and/or worldly success. In order to develop long-suffering you must be able to remain detached from the source of suffering long enough to overcome whatever obstacles confront you. That degree of detachment can only emerge once you've learned to discern the difference between subtle fields with individual qualities and subtle fields with universal qualities.

*Non-harming* is the ability to let go of blame and the will, desire, and/ or intent to harm another person in thought or deed on any dimension of the physical and non-physical universe. Non-harming means more than "Do unto others as you would have them do unto you." It means saying no to the impulse to get even with people who've harmed you or the people you love.

It's important to note that although the elements of good character (discipline, courage, and so on) appear to be separate; the truth is that they are all related because they all emerge from the same spiritual source, Universal Consciousness. That means you already have good character. All you have to do is enhance the conditions necessary for your good character to emerge and to be expressed freely at the appropriate time.

---

### Exercises: Healing Character

I've included exercises to enhance each quality associated with good character. Instead of dwelling on your character defects practice these exercises and in a short time you will receive the benefits, which include a healthier relationship to your Self and to Universal Consciousness, the source of good health and healing.

### *Discipline*

Problems with discipline are directly related to polarity problems in your subtle field. To overcome them, you will use the power of your third polar field, which is the neutral field. By centering yourself in your third polar field, you will free yourself from the push and pull of distorted subtle fields. And you will be able to remain focused and disciplined in a chaotic and ever-changing world.

To enhance discipline, close your eyes and breathe yogically for two to three minutes. Then count backward from five to one and from ten to one. Use the standard method to relax your muscles and to center yourself in your subtle field of energy and consciousness. Then assert, "*It's my intent to center myself in my third polar field.*" Next, assert, "*It's my intent to turn my organs of perception inward in my third polar field.*" Stay centered for fifteen minutes. Then count from one to five and bring yourself out of the meditation. Repeat as needed.

## Courage

Courage is a feeling that is associated with the kidneys. Your third chakra regulates prana in the section of your body that includes your kidneys. When your third chakra is blocked and prana can't radiate through your kidneys, you will experience fear. Without the contraction caused by fear, both physical and moral courage will emerge spontaneously.

In order to enhance your courage, you will perform the *enhanced courage meditation*. To begin, find a comfortable position with your back straight. Breathe yogically for two to three minutes. Then count backward from five to one and from ten to one. Use the standard method to relax your muscles and to center yourself in your subtle field of energy and consciousness. Then assert, "*It's my intent to active my third chakra.*" Next, assert, "*It's my intent to center myself in my third chakra field.*" Continue by asserting, "*It's my intent to fill my third chakra field with prana.*" Take a few moments to enjoy the shift. Then assert, "*It's my intent to activate the minor energy centers in my hands.*"

As soon as your minor energy centers are active, place your right palm on your right kidney and your left palm on your left kidney. Placing your hands on your kidneys will enhance the flow of prana through them both. That in turn will enhance the feelings associated with courage.

Continue for fifteen minutes. Then remove your hands, count from one to five, and bring yourself out of the meditation. Repeat as needed.

## Perseverance

People can't persevere when they don't have enough prana. To enhance your perseverance, you will increase the pressure in your energy field. That in turn will enhance the amount of prana flowing through it. The simplest way to increase the pressure in your energy field is to activate your first and seventh chakras, center yourself in the corresponding chakra fields, and use your intent to enhance the flow of prana through your Sushumna.

To begin, close your eyes and breathe yogically for two to three minutes. Then count backward from five to one and from ten to one. Use the standard method to relax your muscles and to center yourself in your subtle field of energy and consciousness. Then assert, "*It's my intent to activate my first chakra.*" Next, assert, "*It's my intent to center myself in my first chakra field.*" Continue by asserting, "*It's my intent to activate my seventh chakra.*" Then assert, "*It's my intent to center myself in my seventh chakra field.* To complete the exercise, assert, "*It's my intent to increase the flow of prana through my Sushumna.*" Take ten minutes to enjoy the effects. Then count from one to five and open your eyes. If you practice the exercise for as little as a week, there will be a noticeable increase in your perseverance. Repeat as needed.

## Patience

To enhance your patience, you will perform the *patience mudra*. To begin, sit in a comfortable position with your back straight. Use the standard method to relax and to center yourself in your subtle field of energy and consciousness. Then bring the tip of your tongue to the point where your gum and upper teeth meet. Put the soles of your feet together next. Then cup your hands together tightly while you press your left thumb against the outside of your right pinky and your right thumb against the outside of your right index finger.

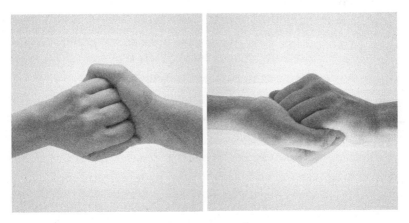

*The Patience Mudra*

Hold the mudra for ten minutes with your eyes closed. Practice every day for ten days and you will enhance your patience significantly.

## Long-Suffering

Long-suffering is the ability to remain steadfast when times are turbulent and/or difficult. In order to remain steadfast, you must enhance your ability to experience joy and manifest it in the world. Your second chakra regulates sexual joy. Your fifth chakra regulates unconditional joy. To enhance the quality of long-suffering, you will activate your second and fifth chakras and center yourself in their corresponding chakra fields. Then you will activate the minor energy centers in your hands and feet.

Along with the two minor energy centers in your hands, you have two minor energy centers in your feet, one in each sole. When they're functioning healthfully, they will enhance the flow of prana through the lower part of your body and help you make progress in the world.

To begin the exercise, close your eyes and breathe yogically for two to three minutes. Then count backward from five to one and from ten to one. Use the standard method to relax your muscles and to center yourself in your subtle field of energy and consciousness. Then assert, "*It's my intent to activate my second chakra.*" Continue by asserting, "*It's my intent to activate my fifth chakra.*" After the two chakras are active, assert, "*It's my intent to center myself in my second chakra field.*" Continue by asserting, "*It's my intent to center myself in my fifth chakra field.*"

Take a few moments to enjoy the shift. Then assert, "*It's my intent to activate the minor energy centers in my hands.*" Continue by asserting, "*It's my intent to activate the minor energy centers in my feet.*" Stay centered for fifteen minutes. Then count from one to five and bring yourself out of the meditation.

If you practice the exercise regularly, you will remain steadfast and self-confident even when times are difficult. Repeat as needed.

## Non-Harming

In order to overcome distorted fields of energy and consciousness that support harmful thoughts, feelings, and actions, you must be able to empathize with other people. You have three fields of empathy within your subtle field. They're resource fields that supply your chakras with energy. To overcome the tendency to harm other people, you will fill these fields with prana and radiate the excess energy through your etheric chakras.

To begin, close your eyes and breathe yogically for two to three minutes. Then count backward from five to one and from ten to one. Use the standard method to relax your muscles and to center yourself in your subtle field of energy and consciousness. Then assert, "*It's my intent to activate my upper etheric chakra.*" Continue by asserting, "*It's my intent to activate my lower etheric chakra.*" Next, assert, "*It's my intent to center myself in my three fields of empathy.*"

Once you're centered in your three fields of empathy, assert, "*It's my intent to fill my three fields of empathy with prana.*" Then assert, "*It's my intent to radiate prana from my three fields of empathy through my etheric chakras.*" Enjoy the effects for fifteen minutes. Then count from one to five and bring yourself out of the meditation. Repeat as needed.

---

### Exercise: The Inner Peace Mudra

Now that you've learned to perform exercises to enhance your character, you're ready to learn an exercise that will enhance your inner peace. Inner peace is a state of stillness that emerges from deep within you. It emerges when movement stops and you can focus your mind on the joy that spontaneously radiates through your subtle field on the spiritual level. The *inner peace mudra* is designed to help you experience inner peace regardless of your personal circumstances.

To perform the inner peace mudra, sit in a comfortable position with your back straight. Use the standard method to relax your muscles and to center yourself in your subtle field of energy and consciousness. Then place your left thumb on the acupuncture point on the inside edge of your right thumb, just below the nail. Place the inside tips of your index fingers together. Your middle fingers are curved inward and touching from the first to second joint. The pads of your ring fingers are touching up to the first joint. And your left pinkie is placed over the nail of your right pinkie from the tip to the first joint.

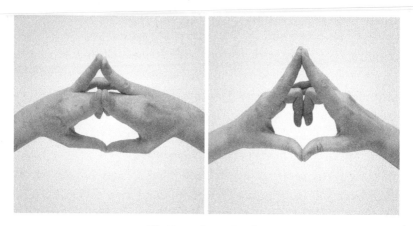

*The Inner Peace Mudra*

Hold the mudra for ten minutes with your eyes closed. After ten minutes, count from one to five and open your eyes. Repeat regularly until inner peace becomes a normal part of your day-to-day experience.

## The Importance of Atman

The region between your solar plexus and throat, including your chest, upper back, and shoulders, is central to the well-being of your spirit as well as your ability to perform spiritual healing on yourself and other people. That is because it is the location of your three hearts.

You may be wondering how you or anyone else could have three hearts. However, as an interdimensional being, it's not as strange as it sounds. On the left side of your chest is your first heart—the human heart. If you move horizontally three inches (8 cm) to the right, you reach your sternum. Directly in the middle of your sternum is your second heart—your heart chakra. Moving horizontally to the right another three inches (8 cm), you reach your third heart—Atman.

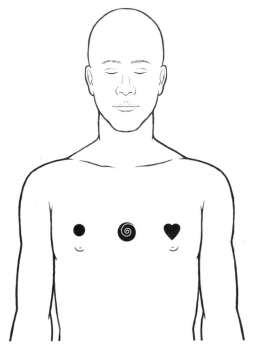

*The Three Hearts*

The Upanishads (a sacred text of yoga) declares that it's through At-man that you experience the liberation of your spirit because it's through this vital point that Universal Consciousness enters your authentic mind and subtle field. This is not to say that you don't receive benefits by stay-ing centered in your first two hearts. It's well known that the human heart can reflect energy. Therefore by staying centered in your first heart, you can experience intense human love, but only when it's not being blocked by karmic baggage, intrusions, and attachments.

Staying centered in your second heart—your heart chakra—will bring you greater benefits. That's because it will allow you to transcend the limitations imposed on you by human love and the attachments that can make it so unreliable and difficult to sustain.

However, it's only when you make the transition to the third heart—Atman—that intimacy and joy will become permanent and you will experience all the benefits associated with transcendence and spiritual liberation. To make that shift, you will perform the *radiant spirit meditation.*

---

## Exercise: The Radiant Spirit Meditation

In the radiant spirit meditation, you will activate your second, fourth, and sixth chakras and center yourself in their corresponding chakra fields. Then you will perform the orgasmic bliss mudra. While you hold the mudra, the next step will be to shift your awareness to the resource field where the universal qualities of spirit emerge first, the third heart field. By enhancing the flow of prana through these steps, you will quickly detach yourself from the blockages that trap you in the mundane world and limit your access to life-affirming qualities of spirit.

To begin the radiant spirit meditation, find a comfortable position with your back straight. Then close your eyes and breathe yogically for two to three minutes. Continue by counting from five to one and then from ten to one. Use the standard method to relax your muscles and to center yourself in your subtle field of energy and consciousness. Take a few moments to enjoy the shift. Then assert, "*It's my intent to activate my second chakra.*" Continue by asserting, "*It's my intent to center myself in my second chakra field.*" Next, assert, "*It's my intent to activate my fourth chakra.*" Continue by asserting, "*It's my intent to center myself in my fourth chakra field.*" Next, assert, "*It's my intent to activate my sixth chakra.*" Then assert, "*It's my intent to center myself in my sixth chakra field.*" Take a few moments to enjoy the enhanced flow of prana through your subtle field while you perform the orgasmic bliss mudra.

Once your tongue, fingers, and feet are in position, close your eyes again. Then assert, "*It's my intent to center myself in my third heart field.*" Continue by asserting, "*It's my intent to turn my organs of perception inward on the level of my third heart field.*" Hold the mudra for ten minutes while you stay centered in your third heart field. After ten minutes, release the mudra. Then count from one to five and bring yourself out of the meditation.

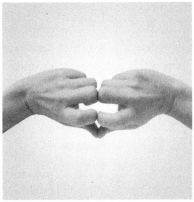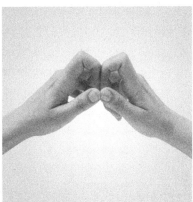

*The Orgasmic Bliss Mudra*

The effects of the radiant spirit meditation will be cumulative, which means by practicing the meditation regularly, it won't take long before you experience the freedom that comes from a spirit that is healthy and is not restricted by limitations of any sort.

---

## Exercise: The Spiritual Freedom Mudra

Now that you've learned to perform the radiant spirit meditation, you're ready to perform the *spiritual freedom mudra*. This mudra is designed to empower your spirit. By performing the spiritual freedom mudra every day for two weeks, you will enhance your access to the world of spirit and you will be able to share more of its universal qualities with your clients and the people you know.

To perform the spiritual freedom mudra, sit in a comfortable position with your back straight. Using the index finger of your right hand, slowly make clockwise circular movements around the minor energy center in the center of your left palm. After circling the palm three times use your left index finger to make three clockwise circles around your right palm. Circling the energy centers in your palms will activate them. When they're active, they will begin to vibrate and glow with subtle energy.

After circling both energy centers place the tip of your tongue behind your upper teeth at the point where the teeth meet the gum. Next put the soles of your feet together. Then place the tips of your ring fingers directly in the middle of the energy centers in your palms.

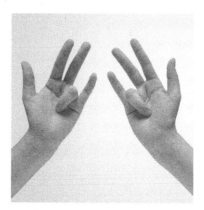

*The Spiritual Freedom Mudra*

Hold the mudra with your eyes closed for ten minutes and enjoy the shift you experience. Then count from one to five. When you reach the number five, release the mudra and open your eyes. You will feel wide awake, perfectly relaxed, and better than you did before.

## Summary

In this chapter, you learned to free your spirit by healing it in three essential ways. You learned to enhance the universal aspects of character. You found a place of stillness deep within you by performing the inner peace mudra. And you learned to center yourself in Atman.

In the next chapter, you will learn to enhance your wellness by adopting a wellness lifestyle. As part of your wellness lifestyle, you will learn how to make life-affirming decisions. Then you will learn how to enhance your relationship to your physical environment and to the people you love.

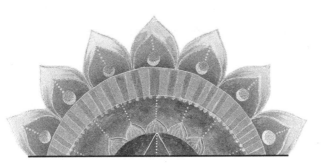

# Part 4
# Restoring Wellness

# Chapter 15

# Preconditions for Wellness

Wellness is a state of radiant good health that emerges from deep within your subtle field. It changes how you feel about yourself, and it changes how people feel about you.

Although most people associate wellness with physical vitality, it's much more. It's both an energetic condition that supports you, your relationships, and the work you do, and it's a lifestyle that is life-affirming and in balance with nature. People who experience wellness are content and self-confident and find pleasure in the simple things of life. They gain the respect and admiration of the people they know because they radiate the glow associated with health and happiness. It's this glow that is the most obvious sign of wellness.

So, what enhances wellness and gives a person that inner glow? From my work, I've learned that wellness has two parts. The first part includes the preconditions that make wellness possible. There are three essential preconditions. The first is the skill and insight to make appropriate, life-affirming decisions. Appropriate decisions are important because they help you to fulfill your dharma; therefore the universe supports them.

Your dharma is your purpose as well as your individual path of self-healing and self-realization. Purpose includes the work you perform and the impact you have on other people. It's by following your dharma that you will learn who you are and what you are capable of achieving in this life. The universe will support you when you follow your personal dharma by removing obstacles and by giving you what you need to overcome life's challenges.

The second precondition is a healthy relationship to the people you love. A healthy relationship provides you with the space you need on the physical and subtle levels to share pleasure, love, intimacy, and joy freely. The third precondition is a healthy relationship to your physical environment. This includes good nutrition and exercise as well as a healthy respect for your body and its needs.

The second part includes the three essential aspects or manifestations of wellness: the enjoyment of your body and physical environment, contentment and self-acceptance, and an abundance of prana in the form of vitality. In this chapter, you will learn to meet the preconditions for wellness. In the following chapter, I will provide you with simple exercises and tips to enhance the three essential aspects of wellness.

## Wellness Part 1: Appropriate Decisions

Appropriate decisions are an essential part of a wellness lifestyle because the universe supports them and because they enhance your life and relationships. In contrast, the universe does not support inappropriate decisions, which is why inappropriate decisions are never life-affirming. In fact, inappropriate decisions are one of the primary reasons people suffer and find themselves trapped in destructive relationships. Nowhere is this seen more clearly than in the most significant decisions people make.

Significant decisions are the ones that have a long-term impact on your life and the lives of your loved ones. These include who you will sleep with, who you will marry, what job or career you will pursue, where you will live, and of course whether or not you will have children.

### Taking the Mystery Out of Good Decisions

There is no mystery to making life-affirming decisions. There are just three simple principles that must be kept in mind. The first is that your core values must be life-affirming and the basis of all your significant decisions. This means that all your significant decisions must support your relationship to yourself, the universal qualities of good character, and the healing energy that radiates through your subtle field. Keeping your core values in mind—and not compromising them during the decision-making process—is essential if you hope to avoid stress, confusion, self-doubt, and the physical symptoms that can accompany them.

The second principle to keep in mind is that decisions aren't made in isolation. This means that all decisions you make now will be conditioned by earlier decisions you made in the past. It also means that the decisions you make now will have an impact on the decisions you make in the future. Therefore, a life-affirming decision should not only bring you a tangible advantage when you make it, it must support your core values as well as your dharma. If a significant decision doesn't support your core values and dharma, sooner or later the decision will interfere with your physical health and the health of your relationships.

The third principle to keep in mind is that when two or more desires are in conflict, you get what you desire most. You may object, but take a moment to reflect on the Principle of Desire. It states, "*Desire is a function of mind. Desire manifests in all fields of activity. Desires that are stronger and more active will dominate weaker, less active desires in all energetic interactions that take place in both the physical and non-physical universe.*" Since virtually all decisions you make are a manifestation of desire and the will and/or intent that supports it, you tend to make decisions based on what you want most, whether you're conscious or unconscious of the hidden forces that motivated you to make the decision in the first place.

You may want to make life-affirming decisions, but if you have a conflicting desire that has its foundation in a restrictive, karmic pattern, it can be overwhelming. It doesn't matter what a conflicting desire is for, either. If it's not life-affirming and you decide to gratify it at the expense of your core values and your dharma, the distorted energy that supports the desire will disrupt the functions of your subtle field and will disrupt your health and well-being.

So, what can you do when you feel compelled to make a decision that is in conflict with your desire to be healthy and pursue a wellness lifestyle? I've found that the problem of conflicting desires boils down to a simple yes and no! You must be able to say yes to desires that en-hance wellness and no to desires that don't. In order to help you say yes and no at the appropriate times, I've included two mudras. The first mudra is the *yes mudra*. It will help you say yes to desires that sup-port appropriate, life-affirming decisions. The second mudra is the *no mudra*. It will help you say no to conflicting desires that emerge from karmic baggage, intrusions, or attachments to other people.

After you've learned to say yes and no at the appropriate times, you will learn a simple exercise that will help you determine which deci-sions you must make are life-affirming and which are not.

---

### Exercise: The Yes Mudra

To perform the yes mudra, sit in a comfortable position with your back straight. Then close your eyes and breathe yogical-ly for two to three minutes. Use the standard method to re-lax your muscles and to center yourself in your subtle field of energy and consciousness. Next, choose an appropriate desire that supports your dharma and your relationship to yourself but continually provokes resistance from your karmic baggage, intrusions, and the patterns they create.

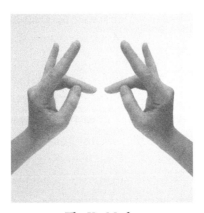

*The Yes Mudra*

Once you've chosen an appropriate desire, keep it in mind. Then put the soles of your feet together. Bring the tip of your tongue to the point where your upper teeth meet the gum. Keep your tongue in the same position. Then open your eyes and bring the tips of your thumbs to the insides of your middle fingers by the first joint.

Close your eyes again and hold the mudra for ten minutes while you enjoy the changes you experience physically, emotionally, and mentally.

After ten minutes, release the mudra. Then count from one to five. When you reach the number five, open your eyes. By practicing the yes mudra, you will support desires that are appropriate. That will make it more difficult for inappropriate desires to interfere with your ability to make life-affirming decisions. Use the yes mudra whenever you have a significant decision to make and inappropriate desires interfere with the process.

---

## Exercise: The No Mudra

Now that you've performed the yes mudra and affirmed your commitment to making appropriate decisions, you're ready to perform the no mudra. The no mudra is designed to deny desires emerging from karmic patterns and intrusion receptors in your subtle field. By denying desires emerging from restrictive pattern receptors, the no mudra will help you to resist, and eventually overcome, inappropriate desires that interfere with your decision-making process.

To perform the no mudra, sit in a comfortable position with your back straight. Then close your eyes and breathe yogically for two to three minutes. Use the standard method to relax your muscles and to center yourself in your subtle field of energy and consciousness. Then choose a karmic desire that emerges regularly and interferes with your ability to make appropriate decisions.

Keep the karmic desire in mind until you feel its compelling qualities emerge. Then use your thumbs and index fingers of both hands to form two loops that are connected to one another, like two links of a chain. Next, bring the tips of your middle fingers, ring fingers, and pinkies together so that they resemble the sides of a triangle.

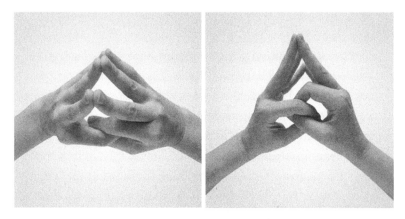

*The No Mudra*

Relax in this position with your eyes closed for ten minutes while you experience the inappropriate desire getting weaker and losing its power to manipulate you. After ten minutes, release the mudra and count from one to five. When you reach the number five, open your eyes. You will feel wide awake, perfectly relaxed, and better than you did before. Repeat as needed.

## Sympathetic Resonance

Keeping inappropriate desires out of the decision-making process is essential if you want to be an effective healer and receive the benefits of a wellness lifestyle. But not everybody knows which desires are authentic and which emerge from self-limiting patterns. To ensure that you can tell the difference between the two, I've included an exercise based on the principle of sympathetic resonance. The principle of sympathetic resonance states that only decisions that resonate in sympathy with your subtle field are appropriate. Inappropriate decisions based on self-limiting patterns don't resonate in sympathy with your subtle field, so they're never appropriate.

By applying the principle of sympathetic resonance to your decision-making process, you will be able to determine whether a significant decision you plan to make will support your dharma and a wellness lifestyle.

---

### Exercise: Determining What Resonates

When a decision you plan to make creates a sympathetic resonance, it will enhance the level of prana radiating through your subtle field, and it will make it easier for you to stay centered in it. On the other hand, if the decision you plan to make has its foundation in a self-limiting pattern and it doesn't resonate, the flow of prana will decrease and you will find it difficult to stay centered in your subtle field. It's these two markers that indicate conclusively whether the decision you're about to make will be inappropriate or not.

If you use resonance regularly as a decision-making tool, it will clear up confusion and ambivalence, and it will make it easier for you to trust your personal insights and intuition. But even more important, it will help ensure that the decisions you make will keep you healthy and enhance your ability to heal other people.

To determine if a decision you plan to make resonates, find a comfortable position with your back straight. Then choose a significant issue that requires a decision. Keep it in mind. Then close your eyes and breathe yogically for two to three minutes. Count backward from five to one and from ten to one next. Then use the standard method to relax the muscles and to center yourself in your subtle field of energy and consciousness.

When you're ready to continue, assert, "*It's my intent to activate my heart chakra.*" Then assert, "*It's my intent to center myself in my heart chakra field."* Next assert in a normal voice the decision you have in mind in the affirmative. For example, if you must make a career decision, you would assert, *"It's appropriate for me to take the new job I was offered."* Repeat the assertion three times. Then observe the condition of your subtle field. Does more prana radiate through it when you make the assertion? Do you find it easier to stay centered in your heart chakra field? If more prana radiates through your subtle field and you can stay centered in your heart chakra field without effort, the statement resonated, and you can rest assured that it's appropriate for you to take the job.

You can check your findings by making the opposite assertion three times. In this case the opposite assertion would be, *"It's not appropriate for me to take the new job I was offered."* Then compare the results. Did you stay centered in your heart chakra field and did more prana flow through it when you made the first assertion or the second? Once you're clear which decision resonated, bring yourself out of the exercise by counting from one to five.

If you're not sure whether it was your positive or negative affirmation that resonated, check resonance at another time when you're more relaxed and more objective. Most problems with resonance can be corrected by practice and patience.

## Wellness Part 2: Enhancing Your Relationships

Consciousness and prana can not only heal the sick, they break down the barriers that make people feel separate. They do that by transporting people into transcendent relationships with one another.

Like an ancient tantric adept, you can use consciousness and the prana radiating through your subtle field to transform your relationships so that they become the foundation of a wellness lifestyle that is both joyful and deeply satisfying. To make that transformation, you must center yourself in your third heart field. Then you must create the mutual field of prana. It's through the third heart field and the mutual field of prana that you will experience transcendent relationships with the people you love. Before you begin, however, it will be useful to look into what differentiates a transcendent relationship from a traditional relationship.

### From Traditional to Transcendent

When viewed from the outside, a traditional relationship and a transcendent relationship look virtually the same. Partners can live together, have children, and participate in the social and economic life of the community. Indeed, in traditional relationships family members can share pleasure, love, and intermittent intimacy with one another. However, the final goal of permanent intimacy and joy, which family members share in a transcendent relationship, will remain a distant dream.

That's why it's important to recognize that a traditional relationship is about living within limitations. In contrast, a *transcendent relationship* is about transcending limitations, which is why transcendent family members will experience a satisfaction unavailable to people in traditional relationships.

To experience a transcendent relationship with another person, particularly your life partner, you must be able to love the universal masculine if you're a woman and the universal feminine if you're a man. That can be difficult because, even in the twenty-first century, many people love their partner but resent or even reject male and/or female power. Fortunately, you can overcome any animosity you might have by releasing the karmic patterns that support it (go to chapter 12) and by creating the *mutual field of prana* with your partner.

---

### Exercise: Creating the Mutual Field of Prana

It's not widely known, even among people who are healers, that partners can create a field of energy with universal qualities that surrounds them both. That field, which I call the mutual field of prana, will be strong enough to prevent karmic baggage and restrictive patterns from interfering with their experience of intimacy and the joy and pleasure that accompany it.

Now here's the best part: the mutual field of prana will continue to connect people so that they can share pleasure, love, intimacy, and joy even when they're separated from one another by great distances or for long periods of time.

To create the mutual field of prana with your partner, sit eight feet (2.5 m) apart and facing each other. Once you're in position, close your eyes and breathe yogically for two to three minutes. When you're both ready to continue, count backward from five to one and from ten to one. Then use the standard method to relax your muscles and to center yourselves in your subtle field of energy and consciousness. To continue, assert, "*It's my intent to activate my thirteen chakras in body space.*"

Once your chakras are active, assert, "*It's my intent to center myself in the chakra fields of my thirteen chakras in body space.*" Continue by asserting, "*It's my intent to fill my thirteen chakra fields in body space with prana.*" Take a few moments to enjoy the shift. Then assert, "*It's my intent to create a mutual field of prana by radiating prana to my partner from my thirteen chakras in body space.*" Neither of you should do anything after that. Just let the prana radiate freely for ten minutes. After ten minutes, bring yourselves out of the exercise by counting from one to five. Repeat the exercise until you can share prana with each other without self-limiting patterns getting in the way.

---

## Exercise: Transitioning to a Transcendent Relationship with Your Life Partner

Once you've learned to create the mutual field of prana with your partner, you're ready to make the transition to a transcendent relationship. To do that, you and your partner will activate and center yourselves in the thirteen chakras in body space. Then you will fill the chakra fields with prana. Once the chakra fields are filled with prana, you will shift your center to your third heart field. After that, you will perform the orgasmic bliss mudra and hold it for ten minutes while you let prana and bliss transform your relationship to each other.

To begin the exercise, sit facing each other with your backs straight about eight feet (2.5 m) apart. Then close your eyes and breathe yogically for two to three minutes. Count backward from five to one and from ten to one. Then use the standard method to relax your muscles and to center yourselves in your subtle fields of energy and consciousness. Continue by asserting, "*It's my intent to activate my thirteen chakras in body space.*" Once your chakras are active, assert, "*It's my intent to center myself in the chakra fields of my thirteen chakras in body space.*" Continue by asserting, "*It's my intent to fill my thirteen chakra fields in body space with prana.*" Take a few moments to enjoy the process. Then assert, "*It's my intent to center myself in my third heart field.*" To enhance the effect, assert, "*It's my intent to turn my organs of perception inward on the level of my third heart field.*" Take two to three minutes to enjoy the shift. Then perform the orgasmic bliss mudra.

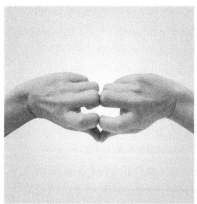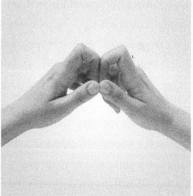

*The Orgasmic Bliss Mudra*

Hold the mudra while you both assert, "*It's my intent that bliss and prana radiate to my partner and that my partner and I can share them both freely.*" Hold the mudra for ten minutes more while you let bliss and prana transform your relationship to one another. After ten minutes, release the mudra and bring yourselves out of the meditation by counting from one to five.

If you and your partner practice this exercise together for at least a week, you will begin to experience the benefits that come from a transcendent relationship. And you will have mastered the second precondition for a wellness lifestyle.

A transcendent relationship is not confined solely to life partners. Family members and close friends can share pleasure, love, intimacy, and joy. For adepts and healers, participating in transcendent relationships with the people they love is an essential part of their lifestyle.

## Wellness Part 3: Your Relationship to the Physical Environment

Wellness has always been associated with decisions and activities that promote physical health and the avoidance of activities that disrupt physical health. Physical activities that disrupt good health include smoking, drinking alcohol, and doing drugs to excess. Inactivity as well as stressful mental activities, such as worrying, also interfere with good health. All of these activities disrupt good health by disrupting the energetic balance between your physical body and subtle field.

Promoting good health and wellness therefore means less smoking, less drinking, fewer drugs, and a less sedentary lifestyle. It also means that you must get more natural. You have a physical body that is designed to interact with the natural environment. And even though life in the twenty-first century may force you to spend long periods of time in manmade environments, it's natural things that have the most positive effect on your health and well-being.

Promoting good health also means regularity and good nutrition. Good nutrition means more than what you eat; it means how much you eat and when you eat. You may have to work in an office building and drive a car on the highway to and from work, but no one forces you to eat processed food that provides empty calories but little else.

Experience has taught spiritual healers that food has an immense effect on good health and wellness. Fresh foods that are natural have the most life-affirming qualities. They protect you against free radicals and other toxic substances. And they contain vitamins and nutrients that will keep your metabolism healthy. Fresh foods also have nutrients that can reduce stress and keep your muscles firm and your skin soft and supple.

Eating fresh food is one part of good nutrition. So is eating a wide variety of foods. No one food should make up more than 25 percent of a day's caloric intake. If it does, chances are you are depriving your body of some necessary nutrients. Chemical additives should be consistently avoided. So should salt. Decrease your consumption of processed sugars. Limit your intake of high fat foods, especially foods high in animal fats. Eat fruits and vegetables when they are at the height of their nutritional value. To do this, focus on fruits and vegetables grown locally and eat them during their natural season.

The human body is made up mostly of protein, which is widely considered to be the most important nutrient. But North Americans need far less protein than they normally consume. The problem with consuming too much protein is that most of the protein-rich food we eat is packed with fat and calories, far more than most people need and far more than you should have to stay healthy. Instead, it would be wise to substitute complex carbohydrates, such as whole grains including brown rice, bulgur, and quinoa, which are often excellent sources of protein, for animal proteins that are full of artery-clogging fats. Researchers have learned that vegetarians who substitute plant proteins for animal proteins have lower blood pressure and far less fat and cholesterol in their system than those who eat meat.

Finally, buy food often so your choice of what to buy and eat is driven by what your body needs. By listening to your body, you will select foods that contain the appropriate nutrients your body needs to stay healthy.

Below is a list of several foods that you can add to your diet. Each has beneficial properties that promote good health and wellness.

**Mangos:** Mangos have carotene, which will protect you from UV damage. They contain zinc, which improves the strength and luster of your hair. Mangos improve the health of the gums and tighten your connective tissue. They're rich in vitamin A, which enhances vitality, and they have mood-enhancing properties. Eating mangos can actually make you feel euphoric.

**Papayas:** Papayas contain large amounts of vitamin A, which will improve vision and give your eyes a healthy glow. They enhance the function of enzymes that promote vitality and other essential life processes. Papayas improve the functions of your heart and circulation. And they enhance the function of your colon, which will enhance the health of your skin and improve your muscle tone.

**Cherries:** Cherries contain folic acid, which improves cell metabolism. Folic acid is one of the most important vitamins a woman can take during pregnancy because it plays a prominent role in the production of nerve cells. Cherries also contain large amounts of iron, which has rejuvenating properties that promote healthy gums and skin.

**Saffron:** Saffron has aphrodisiacal and regenerative properties. In ayurvedic medicine, saffron has been used to fight depression and to harmonize and balance a woman's menstrual cycle.

**Garlic:** In ayurvedic medicine, garlic is known for its rejuvenating and regenerating properties. Garlic can lower your cholesterol level and help your body discharge metabolic waste. It's good for the heart and can be used to fight infections, skin diseases, and sciatic problems.

## Avoid Eating at Night

Although fresh, healthy foods enhance wellness, eating too much or eating late at night can have a negative influence on health and well-being. Eating at night will add pounds to your body because night-time metabolism is incomplete. In addition, your body is rebuilding cells while you're sleeping. If you eat late at night, your body must perform this essential task along with the difficult work of digestion. This stresses your body by increasing your blood pressure, increasing the production of LDL cholesterol, and increasing blood sugar—all of which are risk factors for diabetes and other diseases. In Europe, an old proverb states *"Frühstücken wie ein Kaiser, Mittagessen wie ein König und Abendessen wie ein Bettler"* (Eat breakfast like an emperor, lunch like a king, and dinner like a beggar).

## Regularity

Another indication of wellness is regularity. More than two thousand years ago, Hippocrates advised those around him that regularity was an indicator of good health, and that irregularity both in bodily functions or personal habits promoted disease. Gay Luce tells us that, *"A healthy person lives in harmony with his environment."* She goes on to say, *"It is abundantly clear that healthy human beings are not only internally rhythmic; they are synchronized with their environment."*[20]

The overwhelming evidence seems to point to the importance of rhythmicity to good health, and any program designed to promote wellness must promote regularity. To promote regularity in your own life, begin by examining your lifestyle: the way you live, conduct your affairs, and relate to others. Check to see if there is a built-in irregularity that could be the breeding ground for disease. You can do this simply by spending a week keeping track of the different activities you take part in during the day. Take note of when you go to sleep and when you wake up, when you eat regular meals, when you snack, when you work, and when you rest. You should even note how much time you spend alone and how much time you spend with your friends or family. Keep a separate column where you register comments beside each activity, particularly about how you felt at the end of each activity and at the end of each day.

If you examine your activities for just three to four days, you will begin to see patterns emerge, and you will find that your well-being is directly tied to the kinds of activities you perform and their regularity. For example, you may discover that when you disrupt your normal

---

20. Gay Luce, *Biological Rhythm in Human and Animal Psychology* (New York: Dover, 1971), 10.

patterns of sleep by staying out late, you feel anxious the next day; and when your routine is regular and predictable, you sleep better and wake up more refreshed the next morning.

Your personal experience will invariably validate what the current research indicates; when you follow a regular routine, you function better, feel better, and stay healthier.

## Undernutrition

You can take nutrition and regularity one step further with the possibility of enhancing your physical health and wellness even more. In the 1940s, professor A. H. Carlson and his colleague F. Holzel conducted experiments on rats to study the effects of intermittent fasting on their life span. They provided the rats with a high-nutrition, high-quality diet. The rats were permitted to eat as much as they wanted. The one wrinkle was that each rat group participating in the experiment fasted in different sequences. The first group was fasted completely every second day; the second group was fasted every third day; and the third group went without food every fourth day. The control group ate the same diet as the other three groups, except there was no periodic fasting imposed on them. In the control group, the maximum life span recorded was 800 days, while in the fasted groups the life span recorded ranged on the average between 1,000 and 1,100 days, a 20 percent to 30 percent extension of life span.[21]

Further studies of dietary restriction have yielded other noteworthy results. For example, a number of studies have indicated that undernutrition (caloric restriction) without malnutrition in rats produced chemically younger rats than their chronological age would indicate. Experiments conducted at UCLA by Dr. Richard Weindruch and Roy Walford have shown that dietary restriction has a rejuvenating effect on the human immunological system as well. With advanced age, the immunological system's ability to distinguish between self and foreign bodies becomes blurred, and the aging process is characterized by anti-self reactions as well as a weakened ability to combat foreign

---

21. Roy L. Walford, *Maximum Life Span* (New York: W. W. Norton, 1983), 100.

and toxic substances. It can decline as much as 20 to 30 percent of the youthful peak in old age. Dietary restriction counteracts both of these trends. In experiments with mature rats, dietary restriction beginning in adulthood actually leads to a dramatic and substantial rejuvenation of the immunological system. The tendency of anti-self reactions is also substantially reduced.

What other effects does caloric undernutrition have? Preliminary work with laboratory animals indicates diseases such as cancer, cataracts, skin dryness, kidney disease, and heart disease are found less frequently in animals raised under caloric restriction than rats raised normally. In addition, not only was there less disease, but when it did appear, it appeared later in life.[22]

What does this mean for wellness? It means that fasting once a week, or even once every two weeks, can have a rejuvenating effect on you and enhance your wellness considerably. When you fast, even for a short time, it's important to drink at least three quarts of natural water a day. Drinking bitter salt will help your colon to excrete toxins. You can drink herbal teas as well. Black teas should be avoided.

## Physical Exercise

Regular physical exercise is another lifestyle choice that promotes physical health and well-being. It improves muscle tone and increases mental alertness. By improving blood circulation, it helps release toxins that are responsible for aging. It improves sleep, which has its own health benefits. And it enhances the production of serotonin, which enhances pleasure and helps you overcome the effects of stress, anxiety, and depression.

Strenuous, regular exercise will also help you transcend your limitations, which in turn will help you overcome fear and anxiety. Stress hormones and physical tension will be reduced when you exercise regularly.

For those of you looking for a regular regimen of physical exercise, I recommend Hatha yoga and tai chi. These forms of exercise not

---

22. Ibid., 103.

only provide health benefits, they also help to integrate the activities of your physical body with the activities of your subtle field of energy and consciousness.

## Summary

In this chapter, you learned to enhance your wellness by making simple adjustments to your lifestyle. You learned to use sympathetic resonance to make life-affirming decisions. You also learned to create the mutual field of prana so that you can participate in transcendent relationship with your loved ones. You learned to enhance your relationship to your physical environment through good nutrition, regularity, and physical exercise.

In the next chapter, you will learn to perform simple exercises that are designed to enhance your enjoyment of your body and physical environment. This will help you achieve a permanent state of contentment and that will enhance your physical vitality and connection to the natural environment.

# Chapter 16

# The Three Aspects of Wellness

In this chapter, you will learn techniques to enhance your enjoyment of the three aspects of wellness: enjoyment of your physical body and the natural environment, self-acceptance and contentment, and an abundance of prana in the form of vitality. The first exercise is designed to enhance your enjoyment of your physical body and the natural world. It's called the *morning sun meditation.*

Nothing is more natural and is enjoyed by more people than the sun. And nothing will enhance your enjoyment of the physical environment more than using the sun's energy to bring you into richer contact with your own body and the ecology of life on this planet.

---

### Exercise: The Morning Sun Meditation

The morning sun meditation should be performed outdoors with the morning sun. If it's too cold outdoors, you can perform the same meditation indoors next to a window facing the sun. You can perform the meditation while standing, sitting, or lying on your back. To begin, close your eyes and breathe yogically for two to three minutes. At the same time, let the sun shine directly on your face and body. Feel the sun's rays filling your body from the top of your head to the bottom of your feet.

After you've bathed your body in the sun for five minutes, assert, *"It's my intent to fill the cells of my body with the sun's energy."*

Enjoy the process for five minutes more. Then use your mental attention to scan your body, paying special attention to the body parts that need the sun's energy most. These parts will be deprived of prana and will yearn for the sun's healing rays.

Take note of all the body parts that yearn for the sun's rays. Choose a body part to work on. Then assert, "*It's my intent that the body part I have in mind absorbs what it needs from the sun.*" Let the body part absorb the healing rays for five minutes. Then move to another body part that yearns for the sun's rays. Work on a maximum of four body parts. After you've finished, take five minutes more to enjoy the changes you experience. After the five minutes, count from one to five and bring yourself out of the meditation.

If you practice the exercise every day for ten days—filling all the deprived body parts with the sun's rays and repeating the process on those body parts that need the sun's rays most— your enjoyment of your body and the natural environment will increase dramatically.

## Salt Bath

A salt bath is another way that you can enjoy your physical body while at the same time benefiting from the healing properties of an element that is essential for life and physical well-being. Salt is composed of crystals that can absorb distorted energy on the etheric, physical, and physical-material levels when it's dissolved in water. This means that taking a salt bath can reduce the amount of distorted energy you carry in your subtle field.

In the next exercise, you will take a salt footbath. Taking a salt footbath will not only release distorted energy from your subtle field, it will also be a pleasant way to enhance your contact with a mineral that has been used to enhance wellness for centuries.

## Exercise: Sea Salt Footbath

To prepare a salt footbath, fill a basin with warm water and Dead Sea salt. Dead Sea salt is well known for its high content of essential minerals. It can be purchased at any health food store and in many supermarkets. Then place your feet in the bath and close your eyes. Breathe yogically for two to three minutes. Then count backward from five to one and from ten to one.

Continue by asserting, "*It's my intent to activate the minor energy centers in my feet.*" Then assert, "*It's my intent that the salt in my bath absorbs the distorted energy surrounding my legs and feet on the physical-material, physical, and etheric levels.*" Enjoy the process for ten minutes more. Then count from one to five and bring yourself out of the meditation. Continue the bath for several minutes more. Then carefully remove your feet, dry them, and dispose of the salt water by flushing it down the toilet. Repeat as needed.

## Exercise: Ten Minute Foot Reflexology Massage

There are many types of massage that can enhance your enjoyment of your physical body. The ten minute foot reflexology massage is one of them. It has an added healing benefit as well—it will enhance the flow of prana through the lower part of your body, especially your feet. That will keep the minor energy centers in your soles active so that you can move forward and make progress in the world.

To give yourself a ten minute foot reflexology massage, sit in a comfortable position. Breathe yogically for two to three minutes. Then lift your left foot and place it on your right knee. Rub your hands together to polarize them. Then locate the highest point on the top of your left foot. Mentally draw a line from that point, along the inside of your foot, to the lowest point at the bottom of your foot. This is the solar plexus acupuncture point.

With the thumb of your right hand, press the acupuncture point for ten seconds. Then release. Repeat three times. Don't be discouraged if the point hurts. It's quite common for the acupuncture point to be sensitive, especially if you're stressed.

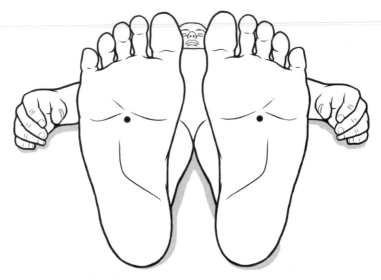

*Solar Plexus Acupuncture Points on the Feet*

Next, use your thumb and index finger of your right hand to massage your big toe. Press the sides of your toe from the base to the tip. Then move to your next toe and repeat. Continue in this way until you've massaged all five toes.

After working on your toes, move to the sole of your foot and massage the bony area behind your toes from your big toe to your small toe. Then massage the outside of your big toe. Continue by massaging the outside of your foot, along the bone, until you reach a point about an inch (2.5 cm) from your heel. Use your thumb and press inward while you circle the bottom of your foot and outline the arch. Then mentally draw a line between the end of your heel and the protruding ankle bone on both the inside and outside of your foot. With your thumb on the inside and your index finger on the outside, press firmly while you make five clockwise circles. Finally, rub your hands together and, with rose oil (or the massage oil of your choice), massage your foot with both hands from one end to the other.

Repeat the same process with your other foot using your left hand. Work on each foot for about five minutes. When you've completed the massage, rinse your hands with cold water for about a minute. Repeat as needed.

## Self-Acceptance and Contentment

Self-acceptance and contentment go hand in hand. The *self-acceptance mudra*, which you will learn to perform next, will help you to accept yourself and remain content with your situation even when karmic patterns and attachments try to coerce you to abandon your values to meet their demands. The mudra is able to do this because it can prevent karmic baggage and attachments from remaining permanently attached to receptors in your body, soul, and spirit.

---

### Exercise: The Self-Acceptance Mudra

To perform the mudra, find a comfortable position with your back straight. Then breathe yogically for two to three minutes. Use the standard method to relax your muscles and to center yourself in your subtle field of energy and consciousness. Then bring your tongue to your top palate and slide it back until the hard palette curls upward and softens. Keep the tip of your tongue in contact with your upper palette while you place the soles of your feet together.

Next, bring the mounds of Venus and the edges of the thumbs together. Then slide your right index finger over your left index finger so that the tip of your right finger rests atop the second joint of your left finger. The middle fingers are placed together so that the tips are touching. Once they're touching, place the outsides of the ring fingers together from the first to the second joint. Then bring the insides of the pinkies together from the tips to the first joints.

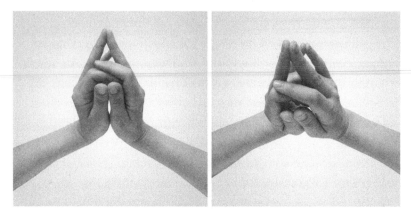

*The Self-Acceptance Mudra*

Practice the mudra for ten minutes. Then release your fingers and bring your tongue and feet back into their normal position. By practicing the self-acceptance mudra regularly, individual fields of karmic baggage and self-limiting patterns will have less power to bend you to their will and to disrupt the satisfaction you get from the simple things of life.

## An Abundance of Vitality

The third aspect of a wellness lifestyle is vitality. I have two tips that will enable you to enhance your vitality by absorbing it directly from the physical environment. The first tip is a negative ion shower.

Negative ions are created in nature as air molecules break apart due to sunlight, moving air, and water. They are odorless, tasteless, and invisible molecules that we inhale in abundance in certain environments. Think mountains, waterfalls, and beaches. Once they reach our bloodstream, negative ions are believed to produce biochemical reactions that increase levels of the mood-enhancing chemical serotonin. It's believed that enhanced serotonin levels will help alleviate depression, relieve stress, and boost energy—all of which enhance health and wellness. An abundance of negative ions in the natural environment will increase both your enjoyment of your physical environment and your physical body.

Even if you can't visit the beach, the mountains, or a waterfall on a regular basis, you can still enhance your enjoyment of your body and environment. That's because every home has a built-in natural ionizer—the shower. I suggest that you give yourself a negative ion bath by spraying your body with cold water from the showerhead at least once a day.

The second tip is to visit natural environments that are saturated with prana. This is easy to do and will enhance your enjoyment of the natural environment and your physical body. Natural environments, especially forests, produce huge amounts of prana that have a rejuvenating effect on people. But not all forests are the same. Old-growth forests are renowned for their ecological complexity and the age of their trees. Less appreciated is the fact that old trees radiate vast amounts of prana into the environment. When there are a number of old trees growing together, the atmosphere around them will be saturated with prana. The effect can be so pronounced that depression can be lifted and anxiety reduced. The enhanced radiation of prana, and the pleasure it brings, will benefit you physically and energetically by enhancing your ability to connect to the earth and to other people. Almost all national forests in the United States and Canada have groves of old growth, especially at higher elevations.

If you don't have regular access to old-growth forests or natural environments, then you can practice the *prakriti field meditation*.

---

### Exercise: The Prakriti Field Meditation

The field of prakriti is a resource field that contains some of the highest and purest frequencies of prana. Like all resource fields, the prakriti field fills your subtle field and extends beyond it in all directions. By centering yourself in the prakriti field, you will experience the primordial form of prana. It's the energy that creates and sustains life and provides you with the strength and vitality to perform all of your activities joyfully.

To begin the prakriti field meditation, find a comfortable position with your back straight. Close your eyes and breathe yogically for two to three minutes. Then count backward from five to one and from ten to one. Use the standard method to relax your muscles and to center yourself in your subtle field of energy and consciousness. Then assert: "*It's my intent to center myself in my prakriti field.*" Continue by asserting, "*It's my intent to turn my organs of perception inward in my prakriti field.*" After a few moments, your orientation will shift and you'll become aware of a large cavity that fills your physical body and extends beyond it. This cavity is the prakriti field.

From your new vantage point within the field of prakriti you will become aware of prana in its primordial form. You will feel it radiating through you freely.

Take fifteen minutes to enjoy the experience. Then count from one to five. When you reach the number five, open your eyes and bring yourself out of the meditation. Repeat as needed.

The more often you practice the prakriti field meditation, the greater the benefits will be and the more vitality you will have to enjoy your body and your physical environment.

## Conclusion
# Wellness Every Day

Any regimen designed to promote wellness must take a human being's complex nature into consideration. It must promote balance and harmony and promote positive attitudes and relationships. That means your regimen must consist of things you will do and things you will avoid doing.

Avoid doing things that have a negative impact on your health and wellness. These could be anything from self-doubt and negative relationships to hazardous chemicals. It might help to make a list of the things that you think have a negative influence on your life and contribute to disease. Then stop worrying about them. Instead, pick out those things you could change with little or no effort and make a commitment to do so immediately.

Next, pick out the things that have a negative influence on your life but would be hard to change immediately. Begin changing them by releasing the distorted energy that supports them. Finally, for those things you can't change, find a way to change your relationship to them. For example, if you drive to work and you're continually caught in traffic distract yourself by learning a new language.

Avoid lumping stressful events and stressful people together. Instead, spread them out and budget your time so you can return to relaxing activities as quickly as possible. Pay attention to your body and slow down when it gives you warning signals such as a backache or a headache.

Of course, it's essential to avoid dwelling on negative things. Instead, find time to do the things that reduce stress and make you feel good. Even if you only have a few minutes, you can practice yogic breathing or take a negative ion bath.

Regularity is important, so be consistent. Start each day with chakra balancing and a short meditation. Twenty to thirty minutes is enough to start the day right. Have a hearty and nutritious breakfast. Try to make breakfast the biggest meal of the day. If you have free time between breakfast and lunch, practice mental projection. If you're walking between appointments, try the exercise the *walking yogic breath*. As you walk, inhale deeply for four steps (taking a deep yogic breath), and exhale deeply for four steps. Keep breathing in this rhythm, without separation between inhalation and exhalation. If you practice the walking yogic breath regularly, in a short time you will find it easier to remain centered in your subtle field and you will experience more vitality radiating through your body.

Lunch should be your second-largest meal, and you should try to eat it at the same time each day. Remember that regularity at meal times cues the body clocks and keeps them rhythmic. Try to take some time to relax after you've eaten.

Daily exercise is an important part of a daily regimen of good health. So, take every opportunity to exercise. Start a weekly workout schedule. To stay in peak condition, you should exercise vigorously (work up a sweat) at least three times a week. However, for those of you who haven't done strenuous exercise in some time, or for those of you who are over forty, begin by seeing a doctor and be sure to take a stress test. A stress test will tell you the condition of your cardiovascular system. Always begin an exercise program slowly, and always stretch before and after you exercise. Consult a fitness expert before you embark on a comprehensive exercise program or pick up books on the subject. They will give you hints on what to do and what not to do.

Dinner should be the smallest meal of the day. Try to put aside one day of the week to fast. If this is too much in the beginning, then start by fasting for dinner one day a week.

The time after dinner is a perfect time to unwind and do a long, healing meditation. It's also the perfect time for the family to get together, so try to arrange a family meditation once or twice a week.

Once every two weeks create the mutual field of prana with your partner and children. All of you will benefit immeasurably from meditating and sharing prana with one another. Not only will it bring you closer together, it will also make your meditations more profound because of the dynamics of the group.

Avoid stimulants and get the rest you need each night by getting sufficient sleep. And remember: to achieve wellness, always strive to stay in balance and in harmony with your environment and the world around you.

## A Final Note

Spiritual healing is an ancient art and science. Those of you who learn its techniques and practice will be stretched to the limits of your creativity. The healer, by becoming a channel of healing energy, transcends the finite and becomes a conduit for infinite love and power. Those of you who have a sincere desire to be healed and to heal others must follow your desire to be of service and to heal. Your desire is your key. Use it to open your inner doors through which your vast resources of healing power will flow.

# Glossary

**Acupuncture Point:** A subtle energy point located within a meridian.

**Appropriate Decisions:** Decisions that are an essential part of a wellness lifestyle because the universe supports them and because they enhance your life and relationships.

**Atman:** The thumb-size spot on the right side of your chest where universal love in the form of bliss emerges into your conscious awareness. By following the Atman inward, you will become aware of your a priori union with the Universal Consciousness.

**Attachments:** Energetic fields of distorted energy with individual qualities that can influence a person's subtle field, and therefore his or her mind, in three ways. 1) They can restrict a person's access to prana. 2) They can create restrictive patterns (personality issues) that are not an essential part of a person's mind. 3) They can keep a person attached to people and relationship issues that remain unresolved from childhood and/or past lives.

**Auric Assessment:** The auric fields play an important part in assessment, particularly on the energetic level for two reasons. 1) The subtle energy that causes disease is heavier and denser and moves more erratically than the energy associated with good health. 2) Like sunlight, subtle energy can be broken down into specific colors depending on its frequency. Primary colors that are bright and clear indicate good health. Colors that are muddy, dirty, or associated with earth tones (browns, grays, and black) indicate disease.

**Auric Fields:** Auric fields are large fields of prana that interpenetrate your subtle energy system on each dimension. From the surface of your body on each dimension, your auric fields extend outward (in all directions) from about two inches (5 cm) to more than twenty-six feet (8 m). Structurally, each auric field is composed of an inner cavity and a thin surface boundary that surrounds it and gives it its characteristic egg shape.

**Auric Healing:** To perform auric healing, the spiritual healer must see, sense, and feel the aura in order to diagnose problems that cause disease. Then he or she must project healing energy stored in the auric fields to the client through the eyes and the minor energy centers in the hands.

**Authentic Mind:** The vehicle through which you manifest and focus your authentic identity and the functions of mind that support it—intent, will, desire, resistance, etc.—into the world around you. It is composed of three essential elements. On the physical level, it includes the brain and nervous system as well as the chemicals in the body, including hormones that influence its structure and activities. On the non-physical level, it includes the subtle field, its organs and vehicles, and the prana that nourishes them. The combination of physical and non-physical elements creates the third part of the human mind called the network. The network includes the connections the mind has to its individual parts and to things beyond itself.

**Bliss:** Is the most powerful force in the universe. Every human being is in bliss, although most people are unaware of it.

**Blockage:** Any field of energy with individual qualities which disrupts the flow of prana through the subtle field and prevents a human from remaining centered in their authentic mind.

**Boundaries:** Surfaces of the auras, resource fields, and chakra fields. Boundaries are composed of prana in the form of elastic fibers that crisscross each other in every imaginable direction.

**Central Pranic Vibration:** Vibration that makes it possible for the healer to channel vast amounts of healing energy directly through his or her hands during the laying on of hands. The central pranic vibration begins in the central cavity of the body. When it gets strong enough, it extends to the hands. Once that happens, the healer can use the vibration to heal disease in his client's body and subtle field.

**Chakra(s):** Sanskrit word which means "wheel." Chakras have two parts: the chakra field, which is an immense field of prana, and a gate that appears as a brightly colored disk that spins rapidly at the end of what looks like a long axle or stalk. Chakras transmit and transmute prana into different frequencies so that it can be used by your energetic vehicles and physical body. There are 146 chakras within your energy system.

**Chakra Balancing:** A technique that will enhance the functions of your chakras and bring them into balance.

**Chakra Cleansing:** A technique that uses prana radiating through a healer's chakra fields to cleanse a person's subtle energy system.

**Chakra Healing:** A form of spiritual healing where prana emerging through the healer's chakras is transferred to the area in the client's body where it's needed most. By performing chakra healing, it is possible to heal ailments in your body, mind, and soul, as well as in your relationships, at their root, in your subtle field.

**Character:** Includes discipline, courage, patience, perseverance, long-suffering, loyalty, and non-harming. These qualities can be enhanced in anyone who has the intent to bring their subtle energy field into a state of radiant good health.

**Color Healing:** A form of advanced chakra healing. In color healing, the healer projects colored rays to his or her client. These rays give the diseased tissue the exact dosage or vibration of energy it needs to be healed.

**Dharma:** The Sanskrit root *dhri*, meaning to "uphold" or to "sustain." Both yoga and tantra teach that all human beings share a collective dharma that is to achieve self-realization. Every human being also has a personal dharma that is his or her unique path of healing and personal liberation. It's by following your dharma that you will learn who you are and what you are capable of achieving in this life.

**Discernment:** The ability to see, feel, and/or sense fields of non-physical energy. With enhanced discernment, a healer can see and feel diseased energy in their client's subtle field.

**Empathetic Healing:** The most powerful form of spiritual healing. In empathetic healing, the healer transcends his or her sense of individuality and reunites with the ultimate source of healing, Universal Consciousness (*see* Field of Empathy).

**Energetic Projection:** Any projection of distorted energy with individual qualities. When an energetic projection becomes trapped in a person's energy field it can cause self-limiting and anti-self patterns.

**Energetic Vehicles:** There are two types of energetic vehicles in the human energy field—energy bodies and sheaths. Both are composed of prana. They serve as vehicles of authentic identity as well as awareness, cognition, assimilation, sensation, and expression on each dimension of the physical and non-physical universe.

**Energy System:** A system of subtle energetic organs composed of chakras, auras, meridians, and minor energy centers. Your energy system supports your energy field. It can be thought of as a power plant and grid of substations and power lines that transmute consciousness into prana and prana from one frequency into another.

**Energy with Individual Qualities:** Energy that evolves and involves through time and space. It can accumulate in your subtle field and create anti-self and antisocial patterns.

**Energy with Universal Qualities:** Energy that never fundamentally changes. It goes by many names, including shakti, prana, chi, etc. Energy with universal qualities nourishes your subtle field and physical body. It has the power to heal, and when it emerges into your conscious awareness it produces pleasure, love, intimacy, and joy.

**Enlightenment:** A state of permanent bliss. In the state of enlightenment, the existential problem of existence disappears and you experience inner peace.

**Ever-present Now:** The eternal present—the space you inhabit when you are centered in your authentic mind and subtle field.

**External Projections:** Energetic projections with individual qualities that one person can project at another. Once you've become attached to an external projection, it will be integrated into your individual mind and ego and become part of the karmic baggage you carry in your subtle field.

**Field of Empathy:** A resource field that will enhance your ability to perform healing. It provides a medium through which energy can be exchanged selflessly without the "I" or the ego getting in the way. The field of empathy has three parts: the Public Field of Empathy, the Personal Field of Empathy, and the Transcendent Field of Empathy. To heal yourself you will center yourself in the personal field of empathy. To heal another person you will center yourself in the public field of empathy. And to use your healing space to heal your relationship to the source of healing, Universal Consciousness, you will center yourself in the transcendent field of empathy.

**Fragmentation:** A violent intrusion of distorted energy into a subtle field. The violence of the energetic intrusion will cause one or more energetic vehicles to be ejected. The most common cause of fragmentation is the intrusion of energy with individual qualities into your energy field.

**Functions of Mind:** There are sixteen important functions of mind through which your power, creativity, and radiance emerge. They include intent, will, desire, resistance, surrender, acceptance, knowing, choice, commitment, rejection, faith, enjoyment, destruction, creativity, empathy, and love.

**Gazing:** To use a strong, steady gaze fueled by prana to enhance healing power and to heal the sick. When you gaze at someone, you will be connecting to healing energy stored in your etheric aura and projecting healing energy through your eyes to the part of your client's body that needs it most.

**Hara:** A strong center in your physical body. Hara is located four finger widths below your navel and about one inch (2.5 cm) forward from your spine. In Japanese, the word *Hara* means "abdomen." Taoists believe that Hara is the place in your physical body where you can find the elixir of life.

**Hara Breathing:** An ancient breathing technique developed by the Taoists. By practicing it regularly, you will reconnect to your strong center in your physical body.

**Inner Peace:** A state of stillness that emerges from deep within you. It emerges when movement stops and you can focus your mind on the joy that spontaneously radiates through your subtle field.

**Intent:** A function of your authentic mind that is active on all worlds and dimensions of the physical and non-physical universe. You can use your intent to program your mental attention to locate a concentration of karmic baggage or an attachment that is responsible for a physical ailment or self-limiting pattern.

**Intrusion(s):** The principle cause of energetic trauma created by the violent projection of distorted energy into a person's subtle field. If you're the target of an intrusion, you may feel like a pin or dart has punctured your skin when it makes contact with your subtle field. The intrusion may also make you feel like you're being smothered or that a wave of discordant energy is pouring into you.

**Jainism:** An ancient Indian spiritual tradition that stresses aestheticism, nonviolence, and reverence for life.

**Karma:** Sanskrit word from the root *kri* "to act," and signifies an activity or action. In the West, karma has been defined as "the cumulative effect of action," which is commonly expressed as "You reap what you sow."

**Karmic Baggage:** Dense energy with individual qualities. In your energy field, karmic baggage creates pressure and muscle aches when you're stressed, and it creates self-limiting and anti-self patterns that produce anxiety, self-doubt, and confusion. It's the main obstacle to the experience of radiant good health and transcendent relationship.

**Karmic Patterns:** Energetic patterns created by attachments and by the accumulation of karmic baggage in the subtle field. These patterns create behavior that is self-limiting and disruptive to power, creativity, and health.

**Karmic Wound(s):** An energetic wound caused by an energetic trauma.

**Kilner, Dr.:** Pioneer of scientific research into the human aura. In 1908, Kilner came up with the idea that the aura could be made visible if viewed through a screen coated with a suitable dye.

**Kundalini Shakti:** Greatest repository of prana in your energy field. Emerged from Shakti via the tattvas, along with you and everything else in the phenomenal universe. It comes in two forms: structural Kundalini and the serpent energy, which is located at the base of the spine.

**Laying On of Hands:** A technique that for centuries has been the preferred method of most spiritual healers. In the laying on of hands, contact is made either with the etheric aura or the client's physical body.

**Life-Affirming Identity:** An identity that has as its foundation self-confidence, self-esteem, and empathy for others.

**Life-Affirming Qualities:** The foundation of a person's power, creativity, and radiance. These qualities include pleasure, love, intimacy, and joy, as well as the qualities of good character.

**Mental Attention:** A function of your authentic mind that functions simultaneously on all worlds and dimensions in both the physical and non-physical universe. With the intent as a guide, your mental attention can be used to visualize the condition of a person's subtle field and physical body. Then it can be used to create new realities of radiant good health to replace the conditional reality of disease.

**Mental Healing:** A technique that includes remote viewing and healing visualizations within your client's body. As part of the healing visualizations, the healer creates tools that can be used to heal diseased organs and distorted fields of energy.

**Meridians:** Part of the subtle energy system in which streams of energy transfer prana from the chakras to energetic vehicles and auric fields. The flow of energy with universal qualities through the meridians enables a person to remain centered in their authentic mind, to form an authentic identity, and to participate in a transcendent relationship.

**Minor Energy Centers:** Parts of your subtle energy system that are located throughout your body. Four principle centers are located in the extremities—one in each hand and one in each foot. Others are scattered throughout your subtle field. Their principle function is to facilitate the movement of prana through your subtle field and physical body.

**Mudra:** A symbolic gesture that can be made with the hands and fingers in combination with the tongue and feet. Each mudra has a specific effect on the subtle field and the energy flowing through it.

**Mutual Field of Prana:** A field of energy with universal qualities that fills partners and surrounds them both. That field will be strong enough to prevent karmic baggage and intrusions from interfering with their experience of intimacy.

**Negative Ions:** They're odorless, tasteless, and invisible molecules created in nature as air molecules break apart due to sunlight, moving air, and water that we inhale in abundance in certain environments. Think mountains, waterfalls, and beaches. Once they reach our bloodstream, negative ions are believed to produce biochemical reactions that increase the levels of the mood-enhancing chemical serotonin. It's believed that enhanced serotonin levels will help alleviate depression, relieve stress, and boost energy—all of which will enhance a person's health.

***Ohm:*** The cosmic sound. It emerged when the universe was created. Its therapeutic effect is well known, especially when it's used with the appropriate meditations and mudras.

**Organs of Perception:** Organs that gather physical input, including your senses, as well as your other non-physical means of knowing, such as intuition.

**Orgasmic Bliss:** An enduring condition deep within your subtle field that is created through the union of consciousness (Shiva) and energy with universal qualities (Shakti). The merging of consciousness and energy provides you with a safe haven deep within you, where you already experience oneness and where nothing can interfere with your experience of a transcendent relationship.

**Polar Fields:** Seven aura fields within the authentic mind that do not suffer the limitations imposed by either your organs of perception or the individual mind and ego. By interacting consciously through seven polar fields, you will be able to consciously experience seven different types of polar interactions with other subtle fields and living beings, and you will restore your control over your subtle field.

**Polarity:** The degree to which your energy field is polarized masculine or feminine. The principle of polarity states that "Everything is dual; everything has poles; everything has its pair of opposites; like and unlike are the same; opposites are identical in nature, but different in degree; extremes meet; all truths are but half truths; all paradoxes may be reconciled."

**Prakriti Field:** The primordial resource field of feminine energy that contains some of the highest and purest frequencies of energy. Like all resource fields, the prakriti field fills your energy field and extends beyond it in all directions.

**Prana:** This extraordinary energy has universal qualities, which means it can be used to heal physical disease, energetic traumas, and karmic patterns that have restricted your access to power, creativity, and radiant good health.

**Prana Bandage:** A tool to heal an ailment created by a buildup of distorted energy. The prana bandage can be used in both self-healing and absentee healing. It can have a profound impact on a person's psychological health and the health of their energy field because it will seal the energetic wound created by an intrusion of distorted energy.

**Prana Box:** One of the most powerful tools available to the healer. It combines the healing power of prana with the overwhelming healing power of consciousness in the form of bliss. The healer surrounds the diseased field with a box made of prana and then fills the box with bliss. Since bliss and distorted fields cannot occupy the same space at the same time, the distorted fields are permanently released.

**Prana Brush:** An extremely effective tool that radiates prana when brushed against a diseased organ during mental healing.

**Pranayama:** The science of breath control. Prana was so important to the ancient masters of yoga and tantra that they developed pranayama. When a person becomes a master of pranayama, he or she can use prana to renew, create, and, most importantly, heal.

**Regularity:** The state of being internally rhythmic as well as synchronized with the environment, which is an indication of good health. On the other hand, irregularity both in bodily functions or personal habits promotes disease.

**Remote Viewing:** A technique used by healers to distinguish healthy energy on the subtle planes from the energy that causes disease.

**Resonance:** The vibration or mean frequency that is the signature of a field of energy or living being. Every living being and/or field of energy with individual or universal qualities has its own resonance.

**Resource Field:** A field of consciousness and/or energy with universal qualities that nourishes a person's subtle field and the energetic vehicles within it. Resource fields are almost infinite in size.

**Restrictive Belief:** Any belief accepted as true by an institution of society that prevents people from expressing themselves freely. Restrictive beliefs restrict the flow of prana and make it difficult for people to stay centered in their subtle fields.

**Ruling Meridians:** Streams of energy that connect your chakras to your subtle fields and physical body. According to ancient texts there are ten ruling meridians. The three most important are the Ida, Pingala, and Sushumna.

**Sheaths:** Energetic vehicles composed of energy with universal qualities. They allow you form an authentic identity so that you can interact directly with your external environment and other sentient beings.

**Shiva/Shakti:** Shiva and Shakti are revered as both the divine couple and as the archetypes for consciousness (Shiva) and energy (Shakti).

**Standard Method:** A technique that will center you in your strong center in your subtle field of energy and consciousness. It takes about twenty minutes. In the first part, the major muscle groups of the physical body are relaxed by contracting and releasing them. In the second part, intent is used to turn your organs of perception inward in order to locate and stay centered in the subtle field.

**Subtle Energy System:** The chakra gates, chakra fields, meridians, auras, and minor energy centers scattered through your subtle energy field. In the same way that an electrical grid provides energy to homes and businesses, the organs of your subtle energy system transmit and transmute all the prana your physical body and your energetic vehicles need to function healthfully.

**Subtle Field:** The field of energy and consciousness that interpenetrates the physical body and surrounds it on all levels of body, soul, and spirit. Your subtle field contains vehicles of energy and consciousness that allow you to express yourself and interact with your environment on both the physical and non-physical levels. It also contains resource fields and a subtle energy system that supplies your subtle field with life-affirming energy.

**Sushumna:** The most important masculine meridian in the human energy system. It originates at the perineum, at the base of the spine, and extends upward along the spine to the seventh chakra at the crown of your head and beyond. The masculine parts of the seven traditional chakra gates are connected to it.

**Sympathetic Resonance:** Having the quality to enhance the level of prana radiating through the subtle field and make it easier to stay centered in it. The principle of sympathetic resonance states that only decisions that resonate in sympathy with your subtle field are appropriate. Inappropriate decisions based on self-limiting patterns don't resonate in sympathy with your subtle field so they're never appropriate. By applying the principle of sympathetic resonance to your decision-making process, you will be able to determine whether a significant decision you plan to make will support your dharma and a wellness lifestyle.

**Tantra:** An ancient school of Indian thought that views energy with universal qualities and consciousness as essentially the same. Shiva, who represents consciousness, and Shakti, who represents energy, were depicted in tantric iconography in eternal embrace.

**Tattvas:** Steps in the evolutionary process. The word combines the Sanskrit root *tat,* which means "that," and *tvam,* which means "thou" or "you." Thus *tattva* signifies the ancient truth that you are always in union with Universal Consciousness and that you can experience the benefits of union (which include pleasure, love, intimacy, and joy) by remaining centered in your authentic mind and subtle field. According to yoga and tantra, evolution in the physical and non-physical universe has gone through thirty-six steps already.

**Third Heart Field:** A resource field that allows one to experience a transcendent relationship with the Self and with the people one loves.

**Three Hearts:** Each person has three hearts—the physical heart on the left side of the chest, the heart chakra in the center of the chest, and the third heart on the right side of the chest called Atman. It's from Atman that bliss emerges into your conscious awareness.

**Transcendence:** The state of union or intimacy with Universal Consciousness, your Self, and your partner. In the transcendent state, you can share bliss and the universal qualities of pleasure, love, intimacy, and joy without disruption.

**Transcendent Relationship:** A relationship in which partners can share pleasure, love, intimacy, and joy without blockages, karmic baggage, or anything else getting in the way. A traditional relationship is about living within limitations. In contrast, a transcendent relationship is about transcending limitations, which is why in a transcendent relationship partners will experience a satisfaction unavailable to people in traditional relationships.

**Trauma:** Every traumatic event includes two traumas—a physical-psychological trauma and a subtle energetic trauma that is non-physical but no less real. It's the violence done to the subtle field that is responsible for the most acute and enduring symptoms the survivor must endure.

**Trishira:** In Sanskrit *tri* means "three" and *shira* means "that which carries." Trishira is composed of the three most important ruling meridians: the Ida, Pingala, and Sushumna. The Sushumna originates at a position in your body that corresponds to the first chakra and passes through the masculine pole (in the back) of the seven traditional chakra gates on its way up to the crown. The Ida and Pingala originate on either side of the first chakra. The Ida works its way up the left side of the Sushumna and passes through the left nostril. The Pingala works its way up the right side of the Sushumna and passes through the right nostril. Both the Ida and Pingala join the Sushumna again in the region of the sixth chakra.

**Undernutrition:** A caloric restriction without malnutrition that has a rejuvenating effect on the human immunological system and enhances overall health and longevity.

**Universal Consciousness:** Singularity that combines all aspects of the feminine and masculine, yin and yang. It is the foundation of your authentic mind as well as everything else in the physical and non-physical universe, including time, space, energy, and consciousness.

**Universal Qualities:** Universal qualities include pleasure, love, intimacy, and joy, as well as truth and freedom. Universal qualities do not create attachments; they support dharma, transcendent relationships, and self-realization.

**Vehicles:** In your subtle field you have vehicles of consciousness and two types of energetic vehicles—energy bodies and sheaths. Vehicles of consciousness transmit awareness. Energy bodies allow you to be present, and sheaths allow you to interact with other sentient beings.

**Yin and Yang:** Yin represents femininity, body, soul, earth, moon, water, night, cold, darkness, and contraction. Yang represents masculinity, mind, spirit, heaven, sun, day, fire, heat, sunlight, and expansion.

**Yin Yu and Yang Yu Meridians:** The two Yin Yu meridians are feminine arm channels that link the energy centers in the palms with the chest. They travel along the insides of each arm. The two Yang Yu meridians are your masculine arm channels located in both arms. They link your shoulders with the energy centers in your palms, after passing through the middle fingers. And along with the two Yin Yu meridians, they form the minor energy centers in the palms.

**Yoga:** Means union. It also refers to an ancient scientific method developed in India to attain enlightenment.

**Yogic Breath:** A breathing technique. By breathing yogically, you will restore your breathing to its natural state and enhance the level of prana that radiates through your subtle field.

# Bibliography

Devi, Chitrita. *Upanishads for All*. Ram Nagar, New Delhi, India: S. Chand and Co. Ltd., 1973.

Hippocrates. *Breaths. Book One [Liber de flatibus]*. Parisiis: Apud Aegidium Gorbinum, 1557.

Kilner, Walter J. *Human Aura*. Secaucaus, NJ: Citadel Press, 1965.

Luce, Gay. *Biological Rhythm in Human and Animal Psychology*. New York: Dover Publications, 1971.

Meher Baba. *Gems from the Discourses by Meher Baba*. New York: Circle Productions, 1945.

Scofield, C. I., ed. *Holy Bible, King James Version*. New York: Oxford University Press.

Swami, Shri P., trans. *The Geeta, The Gospel of the Lord Shri Krishna*. London: Faber & Faber, 1935.

Three Initiates. *The Kybalion: Hermetic Philosophy*. Chicago: Yoga Pub. Soc., 1912.

Walford, Roy L. *Maximum Life Span*. New York: W. W. Norton, 1983.

# Index

## To Write to the Author

If you wish to contact the author or would like more information about this book, please write to the author in care of Llewellyn Worldwide Ltd. and we will forward your request. Both the author and publisher appreciate hearing from you and learning of your enjoyment of this book and how it has helped you. Llewellyn Worldwide Ltd. cannot guarantee that every letter written to the author can be answered, but all will be forwarded. Please write to:

Keith Sherwood
℅ Llewellyn Worldwide
2143 Wooddale Drive
Woodbury, MN 55125-2989

Please enclose a self-addressed stamped envelope for reply,
or $1.00 to cover costs. If outside the U.S.A., enclose
an international postal reply coupon.

Many of Llewellyn's authors have websites with additional information and resources. For more information, please visit our website at http://www.llewellyn.com.

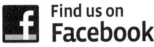
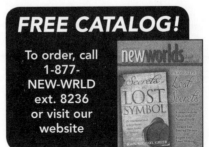

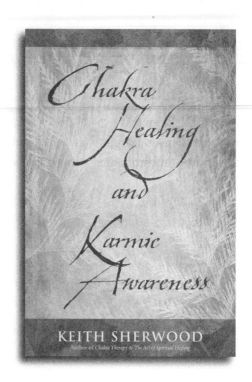

# Chakra Healing and Karmic Awareness

## KEITH SHERWOOD

Author of *Chakra Therapy* & *The Art of Spiritual Healing*

# Chakra Healing and Karmic Awareness
## Keith Sherwood

Accumulating karmic baggage—the dense energy carried from one lifetime to another—is a common hazard for many. This debilitating energy can negatively influence one's personality, relationships, physical health, and spirituality.

The author of *Chakra Therapy* offers a step-by-step approach to overcoming karmic baggage and energy blockages. Keith Sherwood's easy techniques can help you activate the chakras, strengthen boundaries (the surface of auras), arouse the kundalini, and embrace personal dharma. He also teaches how to take care of your energy system and condition it for physical, mental, emotional, and spiritual wellbeing.

**978-0-7387-0354-1, 312 pp., 6 x 9**                              **$14.95**

---

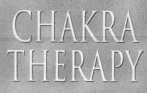

# CHAKRA
# THERAPY

FOR PERSONAL GROWTH AND HEALING

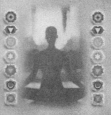

# KEITH SHERWOOD

# Chakra Therapy
*For Personal Growth & Healing*
KEITH SHERWOOD

You are an energy being. Your thoughts, feelings, and actions are energy events—to know who you are and why you think, feel, and act the way you do, you must know yourself *energetically.*

Each of the seven chakras of the human body processes and distributes energy. The chakras transform the energy into sensations comprehensible to us, namely, thought, emotion, and physical sensation. Human problems—spiritual, mental, emotional, and physical—are caused by the inability to radiate energy freely due to blockages in our energy systems.

This practical, easy-to-use self-help book by renowned healer Keith Sherwood teaches you how to work with your chakras to release energy blockages for improved health. You'll learn techniques for increasing your level of energy, and for transmuting unhealthy energies into healthy ones, to bring you back into harmony with yourself, your loved ones, and the world in which you live.

978-0-87542-721-8, 256 pp., 5¼ x 8                                     $12.99

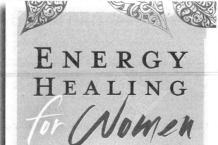

# ENERGY
# HEALING
## *for* Women

Meditations, Mudras,
*and* Chakra Practices
*to* Restore Your
Feminine Spirit

### Keith Sherwood
*AND* Sabine Wittmann

Author of the Bestselling *Chakra Therapy*

# Energy Healing for Women
## *Meditations, Mudras, and Chakra Practices*
## *to Restore Your Feminine Spirit*
### KEITH SHERWOOD AND SABINE WITTMANN

*Energy Healing for Women* is all about healing and empowerment practices for women. Restoring the feminine spirit through knowledge of female energy and power, with practices that focus on karmic release, subtle energy/chakra healing prescriptions, mudras, meditations, breathwork, affirmation use, and even healthy eating tips. Includes story examples, history, theory, and exercises.

- Empower yourself and to express your feminine energy freely
- Increase your self-confidence by loving your unloved body parts
- Use your functions of mind to overcome restrictive beliefs
- Overcome negative archetypes of women that demean you and replace them with life-affirming archetypes
- Enhance both your physical and inner beauty
- Enhance your intuition, creativity, and sensuality
- Make the transition from a traditional relationship to a transcendent relationship.
- Share what you've learned with the your family and circle of friends

**978-0-7387-4112-3, 264 pp., 6 x 9**                                   **$18.99**

---

KEITH SHERWOOD

# SEX AND TRANSCENDENCE

Enhance Your Relationships Through
Meditations, Chakra & Energy Work

BY THE AUTHOR OF *CHAKRA THERAPY*

# Sex and Transcendence
## *Enhance Your Relationships Through Meditations, Chakra & Energy Work*
### KEITH SHERWOOD

Imagine not only having a sex life that's out of this world, but also a more intimate relationship with your partner—and a life filled with pleasure, love, and joy. Blending tantra, karma, past-lives, and universal consciousness, this book helps you use your body, mind, and energy field to reach new heights of sexual ecstasy and create a profoundly spiritual relationship.

Successful author Keith Sherwood shares practical exercises for releasing karmic baggage, overcoming sexual inhibitions, and using your chakras and energy system to experience complete oneness with your partner. Discover spiritual foreplay techniques for multiple full-body orgasms, and ultimately sustain a relationship built on trust and heightened passion.

**978-0-7387-1340-3, 336pp., 6 x 9** $18.95

---

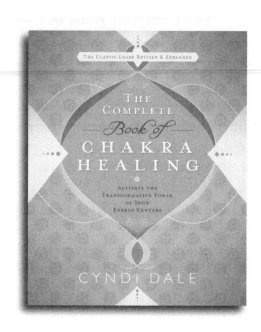

# The Complete Book of Chakra Healing
## *Activate the Transformative Power of Your Energy Centers*
### CYNDI DALE

When first published in 1996, Cyndi Dale's guide to the chakras established a new standard for healers, intuitives, and energy workers worldwide. This groundbreaking book quickly became a bestseller. It expanded the seven-chakra system to thirty-two chakras, explained spiritual points available for dynamic change, and outlined the energetic system so anyone could use it for health, prosperity, and happiness.

Presented here for the first time is the updated and expanded edition, now titled *The Complete Book of Chakra Healing*. With nearly 150 more pages than the original book, this groundbreaking edition is poised to become the next classic guide to the chakras. This volume presents a wealth of valuable new material:

- The latest scientific research explaining the subtle energy system and how it creates the physical world
- Depiction of the negative influences that cause disease, as well as ways to deal with them
- Explanations of two dozen energy bodies plus the meridians and their uses for healing and manifesting

**978-0-7387-1502-5, 456 pp., 7½ x 9⅛**                    **$24.95**

---

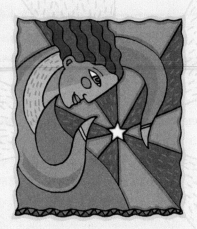

# THE HEALER'S MANUAL

*A Beginner's Guide to Energy Healing
for Yourself and Others*

## TED ANDREWS

# The Healer's Manual
## *A Beginner's Guide to Energy Therapies*
### TED ANDREWS

Noted healer and author Ted Andrews reveals how unbalanced or blocked emotions, attitudes, and thoughts deplete our natural physical energies and make us more susceptible to illness. *The Healer's Manual* shows specific techniques—involving color, sound, fragrance, herbs, and gemstones—to restore the natural flow of energy. Use the simple practices in this book to activate healing, alleviate aches and pains, and become the healthy person you're meant to be.

**978-0-87542-007-3, 264 pp., 6 x 9**                                    **$15.99**

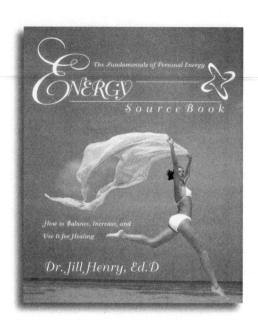

# Energy SourceBook
### *The Fundamentals of Personal Energy*
#### Jill Henry

Becoming aware of your personal energy is the first step toward understanding and maximizing its power. *The Energy SourceBook* can help you discover the fundamentals of personal energy—how to balance, increase, and use it for healing yourself and others.

Experienced in both traditional and alternative healing, Dr. Jill Henry explores four energy theories in depth: meditation, feng shui, polarity energy balance, and chakra work. Energy work is a highly effective, yet easy, tool for well-being and transformation. This comprehensive guide teaches you the techniques behind the theories, offering more than 150 simple exercises and activities.

- Determine your mind-body type with a polarity energy self-assessment
- Unblock trapped physical and mental energy patterns for greater well-being
- Assist others to release their own energy blocks
- Apply universal energy laws to help resolve problems-physical, mental, financial, environmental, and more
- Attract good health, harmony, and balance into your life using feng shui
- Use energy work to help build a more peaceful and abundant world

**978-0-7387-0529-3, 240 pp., 7½ x 9⅛**                    **$16.95**

---